AVOIDABLE CAUSES OF
CHILDHOOD CANCER

Avoidable Causes of Childhood Cancer

Samuel S. Epstein, M.D.
Emeritus professor Environmental and Occupational Medicine
University of Illinois School of Public Health Chicago
Chairman, the Cancer Prevention Coalition

and

Alessandra C. Gibson, MPH, MBA

Copyright © 2013 by Samuel S. Epstein, M.D.

Library of Congress Control Number:		2013909077
ISBN:	Hardcover	978-1-4836-4321-2
	Softcover	978-1-4836-4320-5
	Ebook	978-1-4836-4322-9

All rights reserved. No part of this book may be reproduced or transmitted in any form or by any means, electronic or mechanical, including photocopying, recording, or by any information storage and retrieval system, without permission in writing from the copyright owner.

This book was printed in the United States of America.

Rev. date: 05/31/2013

To order additional copies of this book, contact:
Xlibris Corporation
1-888-795-4274
www.Xlibris.com
Orders@Xlibris.com

Contents

ACKNOWLEDGMENTS i
BIOGRAPHY OF THE AUTHOR iii
OTHER BOOKS v
ABBREVIATIONS vii
PRESIDENTIAL PROCLAMATION ix

CHILDHOOD CANCER

Introduction 1
The Incidence of Childhood Cancers Percent Distribution By Age
 Groups, 1975-1995 3
Leading Causes of Deaths in U.S. Children in 2006 4
The Overall Incidence of Childhood Cancers 5
Trends in the Incidence of Childhood Cancers 7
Avoidable Causes of Childhood and Adolescent Cancers 9
Hypersensitivity of Infants and Children to Carcinogens 14
The Public Still Remains Unaware of the Escalating Incidence of
 Childhood Cancer 16
The Increasing Incidence but Decreasing Mortality of Childhood
 Cancers, 1975-2009 21
Association with Congenital Defects 23
Avoidable Causes of Individual Childhood Cancers 24
Known Causes for Childhood Cancers 38
Avoidable Causes of Cancer in Schools 39
Avoidable Causes of Infant and Childhood Cancers from Personal Care
 Products 40
Unique Cancer Risks from Cosmetics and Personal Care Products 44
Evidence on Cancer Risks of Cosmetics and Personal Care Products 46
Toxic Ingredients in Infant and Childhood Products 48

Cancer Risks of Personal Care Products..50
Cancer Risks of Household Products 52
Cancer Risks of Some Foods..54
How to Avoid Childhood Cancer and Hormonal Risks 56
Survival...58
Carcinogenic Pesticides 59
The President's Cancer Panel Warns of Environmental Risks of
    Childhood Cancer 2008-2009 Report...61
Parental Occupational Exposures Pose Unrecognized Cancer Risks to
    Their Children..63
The President's Cancer Panel Warns of Hormonal Risks of Bisphenol-A....70
Frank Conflicts of Interest in the National Cancer Institute.........................73
Cancer Risks of Dental and Medical Radiation 77
Congressional Initiatives to Protect Children and the Public from
    Avoidable Causes of Cancer..80

CANCER PREVENTION COALITION CITIZEN PETITIONS, 1994-2008..84

November 17, 1994	Seeking Carcinogenic Labeling on All Cosmetic Talc Products 85	
January 17, 1995	Seeking to Ban the Use of Lindane (Gamma-Hexachlorocyclohexane) as Treatment for Lice and Scabies...90	
April 25, 1995	Seeking Labeling of Nitrite-Preserved Hot Dogs for Childhood Cancer Risk...93	
October 22, 1996	Seeking Cancer Warning on Cosmetics and Personal Care Products Containing DEA 96	
May 11, 2007	Seeking the Withdrawal of the New Animal Drug Application Approval for Posilac-Recombinant Bovine Growth Hormone (rBGH) Milk................103	
January 29, 2010	Imminent Health Hazard from Hormonal Meat 108	

PRESS RELEASES AND HUFFINGTON POST BLOGS, 1995-2011..120

*To My Children:
Mark, Julian and Emily*

ACKNOWLEDGMENTS

Apart from press releases and newspaper articles, this book is based in part on my 2005 book "Cancer Gate: How to Win the Losing War Against Cancer," and on my 1995-2007 Citizen Petitions to the FDA.

Warm commendations are due to Congressman John Conyers, Jr., former Chairman of the House Judiciary Committee, for longstanding public health policy initiatives, and my 1979 invitation to draft legislation on "white-collar crime" in relation to industry malpractice. This crime knowingly expose millions of unsuspecting citizens to avoidable risks of cancer from a wide range of industrial chemicals, ingredients in consumer products, and drugs.

In 1981, Congressman Conyers warned that, "Monsanto and the Food and Drug Administration (FDA) have chosen to suppress and manipulate animal health test data in efforts to approve commercial use of rBGH, genetically engineered milk." He also endorsed my 2006 "What's In Your Milk?" book, which warned of risks of breast, besides other cancers posed by genetically engineered (rBGH) milk.

Thanks are also due to Dr. Quentin D. Young, former President of the American Public Health Association and Chairman of the Health and Medicine Policy Research Group, for his longstanding emphasis on the critical, but infrequently exercised, role of physicians in public health policy, and cancer prevention.

It is a pleasure to acknowledge the over 100 scientific experts in cancer prevention and public health, and the over two hundred representatives of consumer and citizen activist groups, who endorsed the Cancer Prevention Coalition (CPC) February 2003 report, "Stop Cancer Before It Starts Campaign: How to Win the Losing War Against Cancer." It is also a pleasure to acknowledge the leading scientific experts who endorsed my 2007

FDA Citizen Petition on hormonal milk, and the 1995 and 2010 Petitions on risks of breast cancer from nitrite-preservatives and hormonal meat.

I would also like to thank my research assistant, Alessandra Elder, for her creative support.

BIOGRAPHY OF THE AUTHOR

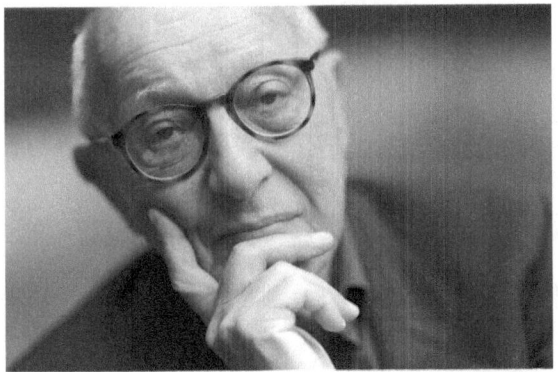

Samuel S. Epstein, M.D. is professor emeritus of Environmental and Occupational Medicine at the University of Illinois School of Public Health, and Chairman of the Cancer Prevention Coalition. He has published some 270 peer reviewed articles, and authored 20 books.

Dr. Epstein is an internationally recognized authority on avoidable causes of cancer, particularly unknowing exposures to industrial carcinogens in air, water, the workplace, and consumer products—food, cosmetics and toiletries, and household products including pesticides—besides carcinogenic prescription drugs.

Dr. Epstein's past public policy activities include: consultant to the U.S. Senate Committee on Public Works; drafting Congressional legislation; frequently invited Congressional testimony; membership of key federal committees including EPA's Health Effects Advisory Committee, and the Department of Labor's Advisory Committee on the Regulation of Occupational Carcinogens; and key expert on banning of hazardous products and pesticides including DDT, Aldrin and Chlordane. He is the leading international expert on cancer risks of petrochemicals and of consumer products including: rBGH milk; meat from cattle implanted with sex hormones in feedlots, on which he has testified for the E.C. at January 1997 WTO hearings; and irradiated food. In 1998, he presented "Legislative Proposals for Reversing the Cancer Epidemic" to the Swedish Parliament, and in 1999 to the U.K. All Parliamentary Cancer Group. He has also submitted 8 Citizen Petitions to the U.S. Food and Drug Administration on the undisclosed dangers of carcinogens and carcinogenic products. These include: talc, lindane, nitrite-preserved foods, silicone gel and polyurethane implants, cosmetics containing DEA, genetically-engineered milk (rBGH), and hormonal beef.

He is also the leading critic of the cancer establishment, the National Cancer Institute (NCI) and American Cancer Society (ACS), for fixation on damage control—screening, diagnosis and treatment, and genetic research—with indifference for cancer prevention, which for the ACS extends to hostility. This mindset is compounded by ACS conflicts of interest with the cancer drug industry, and also with the petrochemical and other industries. The ACS thus qualifies for Ralph Nader's 1975 adage, "Jail for crime in the streets, [but] bail for crime in the suites."

Dr. Epstein past professional society involvement includes: founder of the Environmental Mutagen Society; President of the Society for Occupational and Environmental Health; President of the Rachel Carson Council; and advisor to environmental, citizen activist and organized labor groups.

His honors include: the 1969 Society of Toxicology Achievement Award; the 1977 National Wildlife Federation Conservancy Award; the 1989 Environmental Justice Award; the 1998 Right Livelihood Award ("Alternative Nobel Prize") for international contributions to cancer prevention; the 1999 Bioneers Award; the 2000 Project Censored Award ("Alternative Pulitzer Prize" for investigative journalism) for an article critiquing the American Cancer Society and National Cancer Institute; the 2005 Albert Schweitzer Golden Grand Medal for Humanitarianism from the Polish Academy of Medicine; and the 2007 Dragonfly Award from Beyond Pesticides.

Dr. Epstein has extensive media experience with: numerous regional and national radio programs, including NPR; major TV programs, including Sixty Minutes, Face the Nation, Meet the Press, McNeil/Lehrer, Donohue, Good Morning America, and the Today Show; Canadian, European, Australian and Japanese TV. He has also contributed numerous editorials and letters to leading national newspapers, and published about 150 press releases and 40 Huffington Post blogs over the last two decades.

OTHER BOOKS

The Mutagenicity of Pesticides (M.I.T Press, 1971)
Drugs of Abuse: Their Genetic and Other Chronic Nonpsychiatric Hazards (M.I.T Press, 1971)
The Legislation of Product Safety: Consumer Health and Product Hazards (M.I.T Press, 1974)
   Volume 1. *Chemicals, Electronic Products, Radiation*
   Volume 2: *Cosmetics and Drugs, Pesticides, Food Additives*
The Politics of Cancer (Sierra Club Books, 1978)
Hazardous Wastes in America (Sierra Club Books, 1982)
Cancer in Britain: The Politics of Prevention (London: Pluto Press, 1983)
The Safe Shopper's Bible (MacMillan Publishing Company, 1995)
The Breast Cancer Prevention Program (MacMillan Publishing Company, 1997; Second Edition, 1998)
The Politics of Cancer, Revisited (East Ridge Press, 1998)
GOT (Genetically Engineered) MILK! The Monsanto rBGH/BST Milk Wars Handbook (Seven Stories Press, 2001)
Unreasonable Risk: How to Avoid Cancer from Cosmetics and Personal Care Products: The Neways Story (Environmental Toxicology, 2001)
The Stop Cancer Before It Starts Campaign: How to Win the Losing War Against Cancer (2003)
Unreasonable Risk: How to Avoid Cancer from Cosmetics and Personal Care Products: The Neways Story (Environmental Toxicology, 2005)
Cancer-Gate: How to Win the Losing Cancer War (Baywood Publishing Company, Inc., 2005)
Shopper Beware: How to Avoid Cancer and Other Toxic Effects from Cosmetics and Personal Care Products (Japan: Lyon-sha Publishing, 2006)
What's In Your Milk? (Trafford Publishing, 2006)
Healthy Beauty (BenBella Books, 2009)

Samuel S. Epstein, M.D.

National Cancer Institute and American Cancer Society: Criminal Indifference to Cancer Prevention and Conflicts of Interest (Xlibris Publishing, 2011)
Good Clean Food (Skyhorse Publishing, 2013)
Stop Breast Cancer Before It Starts (Seven Stories Press, 2013)

ABBREVIATIONS

ACS-American Cancer Society
BPA-Bisphenol-A
EPA-Environmental Protection Agency
FDA-Food and Drug Administration
GE-Genetically Engineered
IARC-International Agency for Research on Cancer
IGF-1-Insulin-like Growth Factor
NAS-National Academy of Sciences
NCI-National Cancer Institute
rBGH-recombinant Bovine Growth Hormone
USDA-United States Department of Agriculture
U.K.-United Kingdom

PRESIDENTIAL PROCLAMATION*

NATIONAL CHILDHOOD CANCER AWARENESS MONTH, 2012
BY THE PRESIDENT OF THE UNITED STATES OF AMERICA
A PROCLAMATION

"Every year, thousands of children across America are diagnosed with cancer an often life threatening illness that remains the leading cause of death by disease for children under the age of 15. The causes of pediatric cancer are still largely unknown, and though new discoveries are resulting in new treatments, this heartbreaking disease continues to scar families and communities in ways that may never fully heal. This month, we remember the young lives taken too soon, stand with the families facing childhood cancer today, and rededicate ourselves to combating this terrible illness.

While much remains to be done, our Nation has come far in the fight to understand, treat, and control childhood cancer. Thanks to ongoing advances in research and treatment, the 5 year survival rate for all childhood cancers has climbed from less than 50 percent to 80 percent over the past several decades. Researchers around the world continue to pioneer new therapies and explore the root causes of the disease, driving progress that could reveal cures or improved outcomes for patients. But despite the gains we have made, help still does not come soon enough for many of our sons and daughters, and too many families suffer pain and devastating loss."

---

*   The White House Office of the Press Secretary. August 31, 2012.

INTRODUCTION*

On August 31, 2012, President Obama inaugurated September as the "National Childhood Cancer Awareness Month." His proclamation stated, "The causes of pediatric cancer are still largely unknown, and though new discoveries are resulting in new treatments, this heartbreaking disease continues to scar families and communities in ways that may never fully heal."

However, the President has been surprisingly misinformed. As this book details, the causes of childhood cancers are well-documented scientifically, but still widely unrecognized.

Childhood cancers are uncommon, and represent less than 1% of all new cancers. However, their overall incidence for children under the age of 19 has escalated by 35%, from 1975 to 2009; while deaths were exceeded only by accidents. Nevertheless, the public still remains unaware of the well-documented and avoidable causes of cancers. These are well-documented in the 1975-2009 National Cancer Institute (NCI) Pediatric Monographs Report; the Healthy Child Healthy World reports; the 2009 landmark book *Poisoned for Profit* by Phillip and Alice Shabecoff; my 2011 book the *National Cancer Institute and American Cancer Society* report; and the American Cancer Society (ACS) *2012 Cancer Facts and Figures Report*.

"**New cases:** An estimated 12,000 new cases are expected in 2012 among children under 14 years old.

"**Deaths:** An estimated 1,350 cancer deaths are expected among children under the age of 14, about one-third from leukemia. While uncommon, cancer is now the second leading cause of death in children, exceeded only by accidents and injuries. However, mortality rates have declined by 66% over recent decades, from 6.5 (per 100,000) in 1969 to 2.2 in 2008. This substantial progress is clearly attributable to major improvements in treatment.

---

* Based in part on the American Cancer Society. Cancer Facts and Figures, 2012.

"**Signs and symptoms:** Early symptoms are usually not obvious or specific. Parents should ensure that children have regular medical checkups and be alert to any unusual and persistent symptoms. Signs of childhood cancer include an unusual mass or swelling; unexplained paleness or loss of energy; sudden tendency to bruise; a persistent, localized pain; prolonged, unexplained fever or illness; frequent headaches, often with vomiting; sudden eye or vision changes; and excessive, rapid weight loss. Major categories of childhood cancers, as a percent of all these cancers, and their common symptoms include:

- Leukemia (34% of all childhood cancers), may be recognized by bone and joint pain, weakness, pale skin, bleeding, and fever
- Brain and other nervous system (27%), which may cause headaches, nausea, vomiting, blurred or double vision, dizziness, and difficulty walking or handling objects
- Neuroblastoma (7%), a cancer of the nervous system that is most common in children younger than 5 years of age and usually appears as a swelling in the abdomen
- Wilms tumor (5%), a kidney cancer that may be recognized by a swelling or lump in the abdomen
- Non-Hodgkin lymphoma (4%) and Hodgkin lymphoma (4%), which affect lymph nodes, may spread to bone marrow and other organs, and cause swelling of lymph nodes in the neck, armpit, or groin, as well as weakness and fever
- Rhabdomyosarcoma (3%), a soft tissue sarcoma that can occur in the head and neck, genitourinary area, trunk, and extremities, and may cause pain and/or a mass or swelling
- Retinoblastoma (3%), an eye cancer typically recognized because of discoloration of the eye pupil, and which usually occurs in children younger than 5 years of age
- Osteosarcoma (3%), a bone cancer that most often occurs in adolescents and commonly appears as sporadic pain in the affected bone that may worsen at night or with activity, with eventual progression to local swelling
- Ewing sarcoma (1%), another bone cancer that is most common in adolescents, typically manifests as local pain."

THE INCIDENCE OF CHILDHOOD CANCERS PERCENT DISTRIBUTION BY AGE GROUPS*

	YEARS AGE GROUPS				
ALL SITES	< 5	5-9	10-14	15-19	< 20
Leukemia	36.1	33.4	21.8	31.5	25.2
Lyphomas and reticuloendothelial cancers	3.9	12.9	20.6	10.7	15.5
Brain and Spinal cancer	16.6	27.7	19.6	20.2	16.7
Sympathetic nervous system	14.3	2.7	1.2	7.8	5.4
Neuroblastoma	14.0	2.6	0.8	7.5	5.1
Kidney tumours	9.7	5.4	1.1	6.3	4.4
Liver tumors	2.2	0.4	0.6	1.3	1.1
Bone tumors	0.6	4.6	11.3	4.5	5.6
Soft-tissue sarcomas	5.6	7.5	9.1	7.0	7.4
Germ-cell and gonadal tumors	3.3	2.0	5.3	3.5	7.0
Other and unspecified cancers	0.5	0.3	0.6	0.5	0.6

* National Cancer Institute (NCI) SEER Pediatric Monograph.

LEADING CAUSES OF DEATH IN CHILDREN UNDER 15 YEARS IN 2006,*

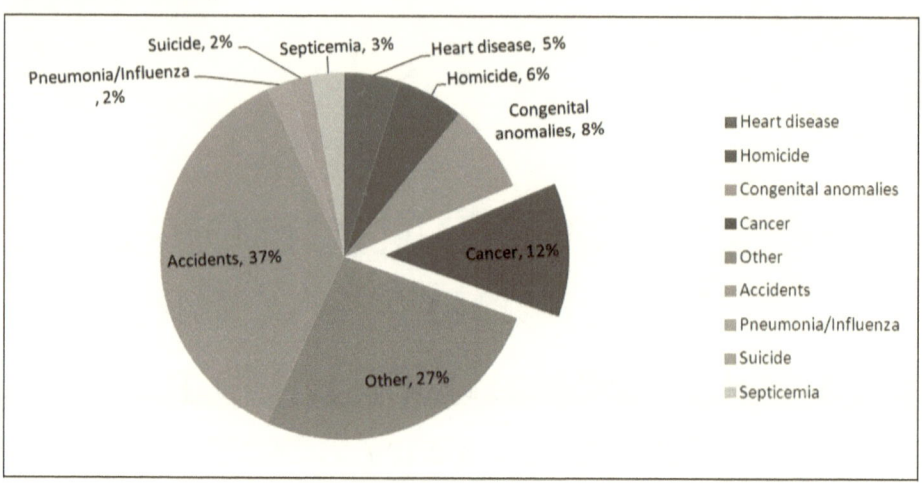

LEADING CAUSES OF DEATH IN CHILDREN AGES 15-19 YEARS IN 2006*

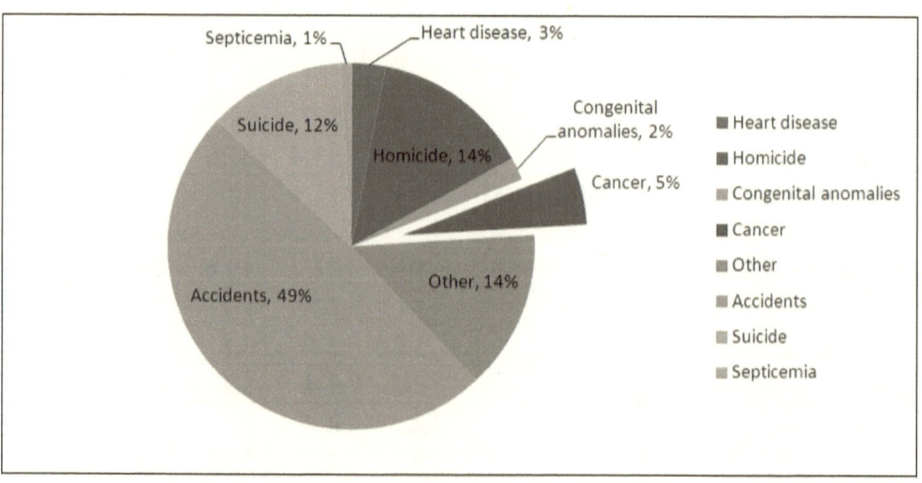

---

* Pizzo and Poplack. *Principles and Practice of Pediatric Oncology 6th edition.* Philadelphia: Lippincott Williams & Wilkins, 2011: Data from the National Center for Health Statistics.
* Pizzo and Poplack. *Principles and Practice of Pediatric Oncology 6th edition.* Philadelphia: Lippincott Williams & Wilkins, 2011: Data from the National Center for Health Statistics.

THE OVERALL INCIDENCE OF CHILDHOOD CANCERS

- The peak incidence of childhood cancers, about 30 per million, occurs during the first year of life.
- Cancers in infancy represent 10% of all those among children under 15 years old.
- Neuroblastoma, is the most common childhood cancer, comprising 28% of all infant cancers.
- Leukemias comprise 17% of all infant cancers, and represent the next commonest of all childhood cancers.
- Central nervous system cancers comprise 13% of all those in infants, with an average annual incidence of nearly 30 per million.
- The average annual incidence rates for malignant germ cell and soft tissue cancers are both 15 per million. Each comprises about 6% of all infant cancers.
- Leukemias account for a substantial proportion of racial differences, in that the average annual rate for white infants is 66% higher than for black.
- The cancers that predominate among infants and young children, neuroblastoma, Wilms tumor, retinoblastoma, and hepatoblastoma, are uncommon among those 15-19 years old.
- The incidence of cancer among adolescents (15-19 year-olds) is 202 per million and similar to that among 0-4 year-olds, but substantially greater than that for 5-9 and 10-14 year olds. Their spectrum of cancers is also distinctive from that in young children.
- The annual incidence of cancer for adolescents increased from 183 per million in 1979 and to 204 per million in 1995. The largest contributors to this increase were germ cell, trophoblastic, and other

gonadal tumors (specifically testicular and ovarian germ cell). Smaller increases were noted for non-Hodgkin's lymphoma, osteosarcoma, and acute lymphoblastic leukemia.
- Approximately 1,050 children and adolescents younger than 20 are diagnosed with cancer each year, of which are melanomas. The majority of these are thyroid (35.5%), and melanomas (30.9%). Adrenocortical (1.3%), nasopharyngeal (4.5%), and skin cancers (0.5%) combined accounted for only a small proportion of the total, while other and unspecified cancers comprised 27.3%.
- The incidence rates for thyroid cancers are highest among the 15-19 year olds, and are much higher among females (24.4 per million) than males (4.7 per million).
- The incidence rates for malignant melanoma are highest among 15-19 year olds, and higher among females (16.5 per million) than males (10.0 per million).

TRENDS IN THE INCIDENCE OF CHILDHOOD CANCERS

From 1975 to 2009, the incidence of childhood cancer has increased alarmingly, but still generally unrecognized, by 34%. However, this increase has been paralleled by a 53% decrease in mortality, an average of 1.5% per year. For children age 0-14 and 0-19 years, the overall incidence of cancer from 1999 to 2008 increased by 0.5% and 0.6%, per year, respectively.

As emphasized in the June 8, 2012 *Cancer Letter*, "Childhood cancer is not rare, only accidents and injuries are responsible for more deaths in children between 1 and 20 years old. One in 300 children is diagnosed with cancer before the age of 20. There are approximately 12,500 new cases of cancer in children and adolescents younger than 20 each year in the United States, with more than 2,000 deaths each year.—"Taken together, childhood cancers now represent the sixth most common cancer overall, exceeded only by the major adult cancers.—More amazing is the fact that very little of the progress in treating acute lymphatic leukemia—and for that matter in any of the childhood cancers—has emerged from the development of new (chemotherapy) agents."

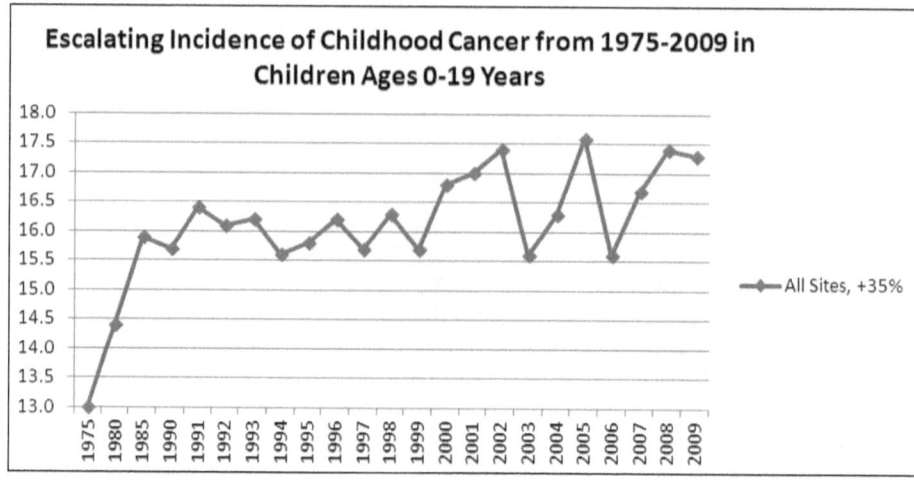

AVOIDABLE CAUSES OF CHILDHOOD AND ADOLESCENT CANCERS*

DOMESTIC EXPOSURE TO CARCINOGENS

1. Second hand smoke emitted from burning end of tobacco products.
2. Third hand smoke (residual tobacco smoke pollutants on clothing and hair of smokers, furnishings, and indoor dust).
3. Carcinogens in flea and tick pet collars.
4. Nitrite preservatives in deli meat, hot dogs, and baby foods. These have been directly related to childhood leukemia and brain cancer.
5. Contamination of meat from cattle implanted with carcinogenic sex hormones in feedlots prior to slaughter.
6. Irradiated meat.
7. Carcinogenic pesticides with environmental exposures from home, lawn, garden, and drinking water, and from pet flea collars.
8. Carcinogenic ingredients in baby bath and personal care products, and children's toiletries.
9. Genetically engineered (rBGH) milk and other dairy products.
10. Drinking water and eating food contaminated with carcinogenic pesticides

---

* Based in part on the author's 2003 Cancer Prevention Coalition Report."*THE STOP CANCER BEFORE IT STARTS CAMPAIGN: How To Win The Losing War Against Cancer.*" This was co-sponsored by 8 leading cancer prevention experts, and endorsed by over 100 activists and citizen groups.

11. Drinking water and eating food contaminated with radionuclides from nearby nuclear plants.
12. Carry home of paternal or maternal occupational carcinogens on skin and clothing.
13. Residence near nuclear energy plants, hazardous waste sites, chemical power plants, municipal incinerators, and major road ways.

As industrial facilities or waste sites are shut down, they may leave heavily contaminated soil behind them. If housing tracts, schools, or office buildings are built over these areas, heavy exposures are likely to result, even in the distant future. Children who play in and around the local soil are likely to receive direct exposure. They may also receive such exposure from former dump sites or industrial areas that have not been reused for new construction. Such sites are often attractive to children because of the absence of adult supervision, besides "play" objects such as old equipment an barrels and strangely colored soils. Major lead exposures have resulted from schools being built on the site of old battery factories; children on the playground picked up lead-contaminated soil and ingested it with their candy or lunches.[*]

"The greatest exposure to many toxic chemicals takes place in our own homes, according to studies conducted by the U.S. Environmental Protection Agency. New chemicals and materials on the market may react adversely with one of the thousands already available."[**]

ENVIRONMENTAL AND OCCUPATIONAL EXPOSURES TO CARCINOGENS

1. Proximity of residence to petrochemical industries, municipal incinerators, hazardous waste sites, or large scale combustion processes.
2. Proximity of residence to nuclear power stations and operating reactors. Childhood cancer, particularly leukemia incidence and mortality exceeds the national average in many of these locations. In 1979, Lyon reported that excess childhood leukemia in southern Utah was associated with fallout from 26 above-ground nuclear weapons tests in Nevada between 1951 and 1958. The observed leukemia mortality was more than twice that expected for children living in high fallout counties compared to control children from before and after the test period. These concerns, besides new "further

---

[*] EPSTEIN, S.S, BROWN, L, and POPE, C. *Hazardous Wastes in America.* 1982.
[**] WINTER, RUTH. *A Consumer's Dictionary of Household, Yard and Office Chemicals,* 2007.

information," indicated that children exposed to radioactive fallout experienced a higher than the "spontaneous" incidence of leukemia.
3. Exposure to carcinogenic pesticides from agricultural and urban spraying, and uses in schools, including wood playground sets treated with chromated copper arsenate.
4. Pre-and post-conception maternal or paternal exposures to occupational carcinogens. Based on a 1986 analysis of 17 studies on parental exposures to occupational carcinogens, David Savitz reported 17 cancer cases and deaths, particularly brain, in their children.
5. Publications in 2005 and 2007 expressed concerns on the relation between mobile phone use by children and adolescents and brain cancer. However, an extensive June 2011 international study failed to confirm these concerns.
6. TRIS ((2,3-dibromopropyl) phosphate), a potent mutagen and carcinogen, was found on unwashed children's sleepwear at concentrations of up to 72,000 parts per million (ppm). Michigan Chemical produced some 54 million pounds of TRIS, a flame-retardant chemical used in children's sleepwear until 1977, when it was banned as hazardous substance by the United States Consumer product Safety Commission. Significant quantities of TRIS could be ingested through children's and infants' frequent mouthing of the material or through skin absorption. It is estimated that over 60 million children were exposed to potentially dangerous levels of this toxin.*

MEDICAL EXPOSURES TO CARCINOGENS

1. Full mouth dental X rays.
2. Repeated dental X rays.
3. Repeated and/or unnecessary X-rays, especially in late pregnancy.
4. Ionizing radiation for treatment of scalp ringworm or enlarged tonsils.
5. Maternal diagnostic X-radiation during late pregnancy, particularly computerized tomography (CT) high dose scans.
6. Maternal endocrine (hormonal) disruptive drugs during pregnancy; the estrogenic DES and the anti-epilepticDilantin.
7. Pediatric prescription drugs, such as lindane shampoos, and Ritalin for treatment of attention deficit disorders.

---

* EPSTEIN, S.S, BROWN, L, and POPE, C. *Hazardous Wastes in America*. 1982.

In spite well-documented evidence on the avoidable causes of childhood cancer, the National Cancer Institute has claimed that "the causes of childhood cancer are largely unknown."

As warned in a October 29, 2009 report in *The Bulletin*, radiation dosage, particularly from computed tomography (CT), escalated from 3 million in 1980 to 62 million in 2006.

A standard chest X-ray exposes patients to about 0.1 mSv radiation, while a computed tomography (CT) scan exposes patients by up to 20 mSv, 200-fold greater than standard radiation. According to Dr. Archie, Bleyer, a pediatric oncologist, this would represent up to 30,000 new cancer cases caused by imaging—each year.

"When a CT scan is justified by medical need, the associated risk is small relative to the diagnostic information obtained," lead author Dr. David Brenner and his colleagues wrote in the New England Journal of Medicine in 2007. "However, if it is true that about one-third of all CT scans are not justified by medical need, and it appears to be likely, perhaps 20 million adults and, crucially more than 1 million children per year in the United States, are being irradiated unnecessarily."

A June 12, 2012 *New York Times* leading article "Radiation Concerns Rise with Patients' Exposure" warns of the harms "that may result from radiation exposure during X-ray scans.—A recent study (by the National Institute of Health) linked the use of CT (computerized tomography) scans in children to small but significant increases in the risk of leukemia and brain cancer—. An editorial accompanying the study suggests that doctors need to discuss the risks of radiation exposure with patients." However, and more appropriately, doctors need to be belatedly informed of the serious cancer risks of X-ray scans, which in general reflect professional malpractice.

HEAVY METALS

Heavy metals pose a variety of health hazards. Lead, in even very small quantities, is a neurotoxin, causing learning disabilities in children, particularly in major urban ghettos, where exposures to lead are high. Lead also produces other chronic toxic effects involving a wide range of organs. Mercury is an even more powerful neurotoxin and has been implicated in mental illness among nineteenth-century hatters, who used it to treat furs; among families in the American Southwest who accidentally ingested mercury-treated seed; and in Japan, where the population of Minamata Bay and local fishermen were afflicted by a progressive neurological disease due to high levels of mercury that had accumulated in the fish they ate. Cadmium, is implicated in high blood pressure and heart disease and is carcinogenic, being implicated in lung and prostate cancer.*

OBESITY AND INACTIVITY

"A rigorous review of more than 7000 studies on the relation between nutrition, physical activity, excess weight, and cancer risk concluded that there is convincing evidence of an association between excess weight and increased risk of several cancers, including adenocarcinoma of the esophagus, colon and rectum cancer, kidney cancer, pancreas cancer, postmenopausal female breast, and endometrial cancers."**

---

*   EPSTEIN, S.S, BROWN, L, and POPE, C. *Hazardous Wastes in America*. 1982.
** PIZZO, P. and POPLACK, D.. *Pediatric Oncology*, 2002.

HYPERSENSITIVITY OF INFANTS AND CHILDREN TO CARCINOGENS

There are numerous and longstanding experimental studies demonstrating the much higher sensitivity to chemical carcinogens of young animals when compared to adults. For instance, adult mice are totally resistant to the carcinogenic effects of aflatoxin, which induces liver cancer in 100 percent of infant mice. Similarly, benzopyrene induces ten times higher the incidence of liver cancer in infant mice when compared to adult mice. Vinyl chloride and diethylnitrosamine induce 40 and 15 times, respectively, the incidence of liver cancer in infant rats when compared to adults. Similarly a related nitrosamide carcinogen induces 50 times the incidence of brain cancer in infants rats compared to adult rats.

As reported in 1989 by the authoritative International Agency for Research in Cancer (IARC), administration of a variety of carcinogens to rabbits in late pregnancy induces kidney and nervous system cancers in their offspring. Prenatal exposure of rats to diethylstilbestrol, a synthetic estrogenic-type hormone known to be a potent carcinogen since the 1940's, induces vaginal and cervical cancers in their young female progeny. This is strikingly consistent with the diagnosis from 1971 onwards of rare vaginal cancers in young girls whose mothers were treated during pregnancy with the same hormone for "complications of pregnancy," allegedly due to hormonal deficiency.

Some 30 U.S. and international studies have confirmed the high incidence of cancers in children whose parents were exposed to a variety of chemical carcinogens in the workplace during pregnancy. Also, an increased incidence of brain cancer and leukemia has been reported in children whose mothers were exposed to nitrosamine carcinogens in nitrite-preserved meats during pregnancy. These findings are relevant to the striking 35 percent increase in the incidence of childhood cancers since 1950, and the 20 percent increase in the incidence of brain and nervous system cancers since 1973. A 1989 report by the Natural Resources Defense Council concluded that a high percentage of U.S. preschool children are likely to develop cancer in later life as a result of consumption of fruits and vegetables commonly contaminated by some eight pesticides.

In an August 2000 report to the Green Audit, Chris Busby reported "significantly and startling high rates of brain and thyroid cancer, leukemia, lymphomas and other sites in children age 0-4 in North Wales coastal areas. These were all located in the vicinity of the Hinkley Point, Somerset nuclear power station. This finding is consistent with a 1996 report of excess rates of childhood leukemia in France and Germany, besides Russia, 5 years following the Chernobyl nuclear plant disaster. The increased incidence of childhood cancers near nuclear facilities has also been reported in England, Germany, France, and Russia.

Numerous reports have documented excess cancer rates under the age of 14 living near nuclear plants. This includes one by Mangano and colleagues based on 14 nuclear plants in 49 counties in the eastern U.S.

The increased susceptibility of infants and young children to a wide range of carcinogens has been fully recognized for well over two decades. This reflects limited physiological capability to detoxify chemical carcinogens due to their immature liver enzymes. Another reason for the increased susceptibility of infants and young children is due to the fact that their cells are dividing more rapidly than adults. Thus, there is a greater probability that carcinogens will cause DNA mutations in cells of the young and initiate the development of delayed cancers in adult life.

While the hypersensitivity of children to carcinogens has long been recognized, surprisingly this does not extend to their avoidable carcinogenic exposures from numerous carcinogens in common CPCPs such as shampoos and lotions. This was revealingly illustrated in 1994 when *Child Magazine* selected a book entitled *Raising Children Toxic Free* by Drs. Needleman and Landrigan as "One of the Ten Best Parenting Books of the Year." Although these authors are leading pediatricians and experts on toxic chemicals, they ignore the toxic and carcinogenic risks of personal care products, except for a brief reference to lead hair dyes.

THE PUBLIC STILL REMAINS UNAWARE OF THE ESCALATING INCIDENCE OF CHILDHOOD CANCER

From 1975 to 2009, the incidence of childhood cancers has escalated to alarming proportions. Childhood cancers overall have increased by 35 percent, to 9,000 annually: acute lymphocytic leukemia, 63 percent; kidney cancer, 60 percent; brain and bone cancer, 43 percent each; and leukemia, 40 percent. Although uncommon, cancer is now the second leading cause of death in children, with 1,340 deaths this year, second only to accidents.

Both the National Cancer Institute (NCI) and the American Cancer Society (ACS) have failed to warn the public of the increasing incidence of childhood cancer. Furthermore, the NCI claims that: **"The causes of childhood cancers are largely unknown,"** while the ACS frankly ignores their causes. This is contrary to substantial scientific evidence on their avoidable causes, the wide range of carcinogens to which fetuses, infants, and children are exposed, and their much greater vulnerability than adults. Additionally, most carcinogens cause other toxic effects, notably hormonal (endocrine disruptive), neurological, and immunological.

The avoidable exposures of the fetus, infants, and children to well documented carcinogens, fall into 5 major categories:

1. *Environmental and Occupational Pollutants*

A wide range of reports dating back to the 1970's have incriminated paternal, and to a lesser extent maternal, exposures to occupational carcinogens and pediatric cancers. Other reports have also incriminated proximity of residence to nuclear reactors with exposure to radioactive emissions by inhalation besides by contamination of local food and drinking water.

- Numerous studies have shown strong associations between childhood cancers, particularly brain cancer, non-Hodgkin's lymphoma and leukemia, and exposures to pesticides from uses in the home, including pet flea collars, lawn and garden, and schools.
- Pesticides: propoxur and tetrachlorovinphos (TCVP), are both dangerous pesticides. They are carcinogenic (cancer-causing) common ingredients in flea and tick pet collars, and used for urban spraying, and for treating wood playground sets in schools. They are also recognized contaminants in drinking water.
- Petrochemical and other industrial pollutants: atmospheric emissions; contaminants in drinking water.
- Combustion pollutants: power plants; incinerator stacks; diesel exhaust.
- Radioactive pollutants: atmospheric emissions from nuclear reactors; contaminants in drinking water.
- Occupational carcinogens: Over 20 U.S. and international studies have incriminated paternal and maternal exposures (pre-conception, during conception and post-conception) to a wide range of occupational carcinogens as major causes of childhood cancer, incidence and mortality. These cancer include: acute lymphocytic leukemia, and non-hodgkin's lymphoma.

2. *Domestic: Indoor Air Pollution*

- Chronic household exposure to second hand parental tobacco smoke from burning cigarettes and pipes, and from exhaled smoke.
- Third hand smoke from domestic tobacco smoke absorbed on clothing, furniture, and dust.
- Carcinogenic pesticides in the home, lawn and pet flea collars, and contaminants in non-organic food.
- Carcinogenic ingredients and contaminants in lotions and shampoos.
- Proximity of residence to hazardous industrial waste sites, chemical and power plants, and municipal incinerators.
- Proximity of residence to nuclear power plants, as reported in the U.S. and internationally, with particular reference to excesses of childhood leukemia and thyroid cancer.

3. *Medical Radiation*

   - Treatment of childhood tinea capitis (ringworm) with radiation
   - Maternal radiation: diagnostic X-rays in late pregnancy is strongly associated with excess risks of childhood leukemia.
   - Whole body X-rays of premature babies and infants, known as "baby grams."
   - Diagnostic radiation: "low dose" medical X-rays of infants and children.
   - Diagnostic radiation: high dose CT (computerized tomography) X-rays of the head of infants and young children, following a major head injury, has been recently associated with increased risks of brain cancer and leukemia in childhood or young adults.

4. *Prescription Drugs*

   - Pediatric: Use of lindane, a potent carcinogen in shampoos for treating lice and scabies, infesting about six million children annually, is associated with major risks of brain cancer; lindane is readily absorbed through the skin.
   - Pediatric: Treatment of children with Ritalin for "Attention Deficit Disorders" poses risks of cancer, in the absence of informed parental consent. Ritalin has been shown to induce highly aggressive rare liver cancers in rodents at doses comparable to those prescribed to children.
   - Drugs prescribed during pregnancy: the estrogenic diethylstilbestrol (DES); the anti-epileptic Dilantin.

5. *Dietary*

   - There is substantial evidence on the risks of brain cancer and leukemia in children from frequent consumption of nitrite-dyed hot dogs; consumption during pregnancy has been similarly incriminated. Nitrites, added to meat for coloring purposes, have been shown to react with natural chemicals in meat (amines) to form a potent carcinogenic nitrosamine.
   - Consumption of non-organic fruits and vegetables, particularly in baby food, contaminated with high concentrations of multiple residues of carcinogenic pesticides, poses major risks of childhood cancer, besides delayed cancers in adult life.

The Indifference to Cancer Prevention by the National Cancer Institute (NCI) and American Cancer Society (ACS)

The continuing silence of the NCI, besides that of the "charitable" American Cancer Society (ACS), on well-documented causes of childhood cancer is criminal. It also explicitly violates the charge of the 1971 National Cancer Act, launching President Nixon's War Against Cancer, "to disseminate cancer information to the public." This silence is also contrary to NCI's 1998 Congressional testimony that it had developed a public registry of avoidable carcinogens. Not surprisingly, the media remain as uninformed as the public. An April 1, 2003 New York Times article, "Success Stories Abound in Efforts to Prevent and Control Cancer," stated that while amazing progress has been made in treating childhood cancers, "their causes remain a mystery."

Besides the NCI's minimal priority to avoidable causes of childhood cancer, it has failed to provide any scientific guidance to regulatory agencies, as reflected in their inconsistent and questionable policies. This is well illustrated in the current proposal of the Scientific Advisory Board of the Environmental Protection Agency to develop new guidelines for regulating risks "from Early-Life Exposure to Carcinogens."

The minimal priorities of the NCI for research and providing the public with information on avoidable causes of childhood cancers reflect imbalanced policies, and not lack of resources. NCI's annual budget has increased some 25-fold, from $200 million in 1972 to $5.2 billion, since passage of the 1971 National Cancer Act. NCI expenditures on prevention of avoidable causes of cancer have been generously estimated as under 4 percent of its budget.

It is of particular significance that the cancer establishment ignored the continuing increase in the incidence of childhood cancer in its heavily promoted, but highly arguable, March 1998 "claim to have reversed an almost 20-year trend of increasing cancer cases."

The failure of the NCI to warn of these avoidable cancer risks reflects mindsets fixated on damage control—screening, diagnosis, and treatment—and basic genetic research, with indifference to primary prevention, as defined by research and public education on avoidable causes of cancer.

It should be particularly stressed that fetuses, infants and children are much more vulnerable and sensitive to toxic and carcinogenic exposures than are adults. It should also be recognized that the majority of carcinogens also induce other chronic toxic effects, especially in fetuses, infants and children. These include endocrine disruptive and reproductive, haematological, immunological and genetic, for which there are no available incidence trend data comparable to those for cancer.

The continued silence of the NCI on avoidable causes of childhood, besides a wide range of other, cancers is in flagrant denial of the specific charge of the 1971 National Cancer Act "to disseminate cancer information to the public." As seriously, this silence is a denial of the public's inalienable democratic right-to-know of information directly impacting on their health and lives, and of their right to influence public policy.

In his classic 1982 book, *America the Promised*, Lewis Regenstein warned, "Cancer-causing chemicals commonly found in the fat tissue of Americans include aldrin, chlordane, DDT, dieldrin, dioxin, benzene hexachloride (BHC), endrin, heptachlor, mirex and PCB's, all of which have been banned for all or major uses.—Because toxic chemicals are stored in human fat tissue, they become highly concentrated in mother's milk. Its tragic contamination has been dramatized by The Ecology Center in Berkeley, California, which issued a poster of a nude and pregnant woman with a label on her breasts reading, '*Caution*: keep out of reach of children.' There is more truth than humor in this warning. Since mother's milk is often an infant's only source of food, the baby ingests a much larger portion of these and other chlorinated hydrocarbon pesticides on a body-weight basis than does an adult, and the effects could thus be much more serious. The World Health Organization (WHO) has estimated the levels at which chemicals may be consumed without causing serious harm. These Acceptable Daily Intake (AI) levels are regularly equaled or exceeded by nursing infants in the United States."

THE INCREASING INCIDENCE BUT DECREASING MORTALITY RATES OF MAJOR CHILDHOOD CANCERS, 1975-2009[*]

SITE	% Increase Incidence	% Decrease Mortality[**]
Overall	35	53
Acute Lymphocytic Leukemia	58	70
Bone & Joint	57	33
Brain & Nervous System	52	33
Non-Hodgkin Lymphoma	40	75
Leukemia	33	65
Kidney (Wilm's Tumor)	20	0

[*] National Cancer Institute, *Surveillance, Epidemiology and End Results*, 2011.

[**] The striking decrease in mortality reflects the National Cancer Institute's success in developing pediatric clinical trial cooperative groups in 2000. (*The Cancer Letter*, June 8, 2012).

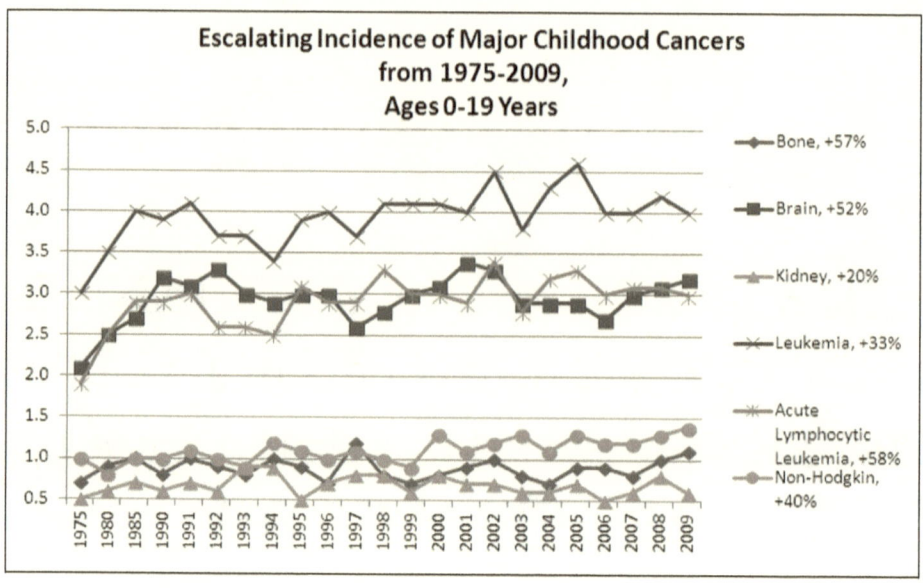

ASSOCIATION WITH CONGENITAL DEFECTS

Several childhood cancers occur so early in life that they must have originated during fetal life, or shortly thereafter.[*] These include acute lymphocytic leukemia, neuroblastoma,[**] and kidney and liver cancers. Cancer in the mother, particularly melanoma, can spread to the infant.

---

[*] MILLER, R.W. *Journal of the National Cancer Institute.* 40; 1079-1085, 1968.
[**] The author is a survivor of this cancer.

AVOIDABLE CAUSES OF MAJOR CHILDHOOD CANCERS

The SEER Pediatric Monograph reported on "Cancer Incidence and Survival among Children and Adolescents 1975-1995," and on "Current Knowledge on Their Causes."

KIDNEY CANCERS

Incidence

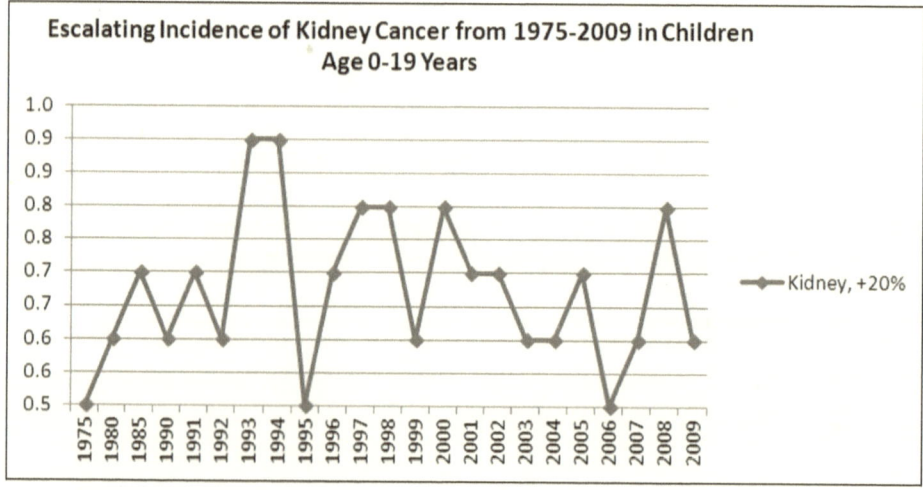

- Malignancies of the kidney (renal cancers) represented 6.3% of cancer diagnoses among children younger than 15 years of age (incidence 7.9 per million) and 4.4% of cancer diagnoses for children

- and adolescents younger than 20 years of age (incidence of 6.2 per million).
- In the US approximately 550 children and adolescents younger than 20 years of age are diagnosed with renal tumors each year, of which approximately 500 are Wilms' tumor.
- Wilms' tumor was by far the most common form of renal cancer in children younger than 15 years of age, representing approximately 95% of diagnoses. Much less common were rhabdoid tumors of the kidney (1% of renal cancers) and clear cell sarcoma of the kidney (1.6% of renal cancers). Renal carcinomas, the most common form of renal cancer in adults, represented only 2.6% of renal cancers in children younger than 15 years of age.
- Wilms' tumor occurred most commonly among children younger than 5 years of age, with very low incidence for 10-14 and 15-19 year olds. The highest incidence for Wilms' tumor was in the first 2 years of life, followed by steadily decreasing rates with increasing age.
- Rhabdoid tumor of the kidney was diagnosed primarily in infants, while clear cell sarcoma of the kidney was diagnosed primarily during the first 4 years of life. Renal carcinomas, by contrast, occurred with highest incidence among 15-19 year olds.
- Females had slightly higher incidence than males for Wilms' tumor during the period 1975-95. For the recent period of 1990-95, however, incidence rates were similar by sex.
- Black children had somewhat higher incidence for Wilms' tumor than white children for the period 1975-95. For the time periods 1986-89 and 1990-95, however, incidence rates by race were similar.
- The incidence in Asiatics is about half that in black and whites.
- Incidence of Wilms' tumor showed neither substantial increases nor decreases during the 21-year period from 1975 to 1995.

Survival

- The overall relative 5-year survival rate for children with Wilms' tumor was approximately 92% for cases diagnosed from 1985-94, an improvement from the 81% survival rate for cases diagnosed from 1975-84. Survival rates were slightly higher for females than males and for black than for white children.

Risk factors

- Certain congenital anomalies and genetic conditions increase susceptibility for Wilms' tumor. Suggestive, although not conclusive, data indicate that certain paternal occupations may be associated with increased Wilms' tumor risk.
- The risks are congenital genitourinary anomalies, such as childhood kidney, genitourinary abnormalities, and mental retardation.

BRAIN CANCERS

Incidence

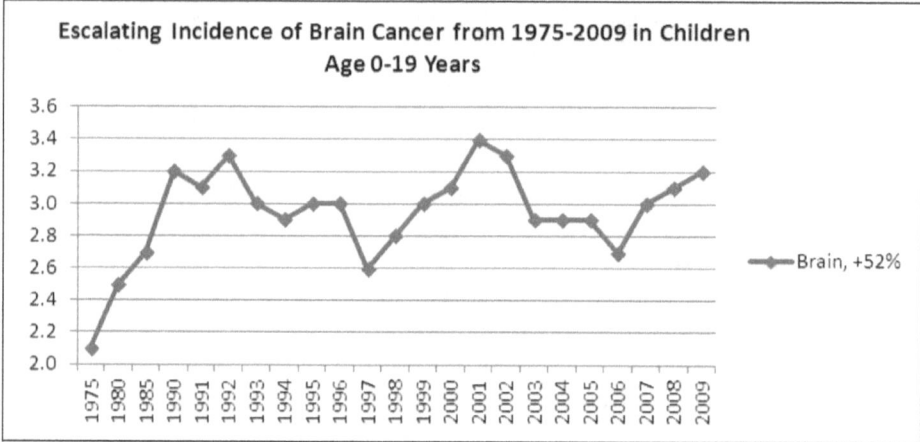

- The CNS malignancies represented 16.6% of all malignancies during childhood (including adolescence). CNS cancer as a group was the second most frequent malignancy of childhood and the most common of the solid tumors. In the US approximately 2,200 children younger than 20 years of age are diagnosed annually with invasive CNS tumors.
- Astrocytomas accounted for 52% of CNS malignancies, PNET comprised 21%, other gliomas 15% and ependymomas an additional 9%.
- Unlike adults and older children, young children have a relatively high occurrence of malignancies in the cerebellum and the brain stem. In fact, in children younger than 10 years of age, brain stem malignancies were nearly as common as cerebral malignancies, and

- cerebellum malignancies were far more common than cerebral malignancies.
- The incidence of invasive CNS tumors was higher in males than females and higher among white children than black children.
- The average annual incidence of CNS cancer varied only slightly by age of diagnosis from infancy (36.2 per million) through age 7 years (35.2 per million). From age 7 to 10, a 40% drop in the incidence rate (to 21.0 per million) was observed. CNS cancer rates were fairly consistent among children aged 11 through 17 years, until another substantial decrease occurred at age 18.
- The increase in CNS cancer rates in the past two decades has been the subject of numerous reports. One concern is that changes in environmental exposures may be responsible for the increasing incidence rates, although epidemiologic evidence to support this hypothesis currently is lacking. An alternative explanation is that improvements in diagnostic technology and case ascertainment may be contributing to the increasing trend.
- The incidence of brain (medulloblastoma and ependymomas) is higher in male than female children. The known "risk factors" for both cancers are male sex and past treatment of radiation to the head.

Survival

- In general, children with CNS cancer do not share the favorable prognosis of those with many other common pediatric neoplasms.
- Very young children with CNS cancer, especially infants with ependymoma or PNET, had low survival rates.

Risk factors

- There is no specific risk factor that explains a substantial proportion of brain tumor occurrence, but there are a couple of factors that explain a small proportion.
- Higher in males than females
- Family history of brain cancer
- Father's occupation
- Pesticides
- Family history of epilepsy
- Family history of mental retardation
- Parent or sibling with brain cancer

- Congenital genetic conditions such as neurofibroma and Li Fraumeni syndrome
- Radiation of scalp for treatment of tinea capitis (ringworm), neurofibromatosis, and Li-Fraumeni syndrome

LEUKEMIA

Incidence

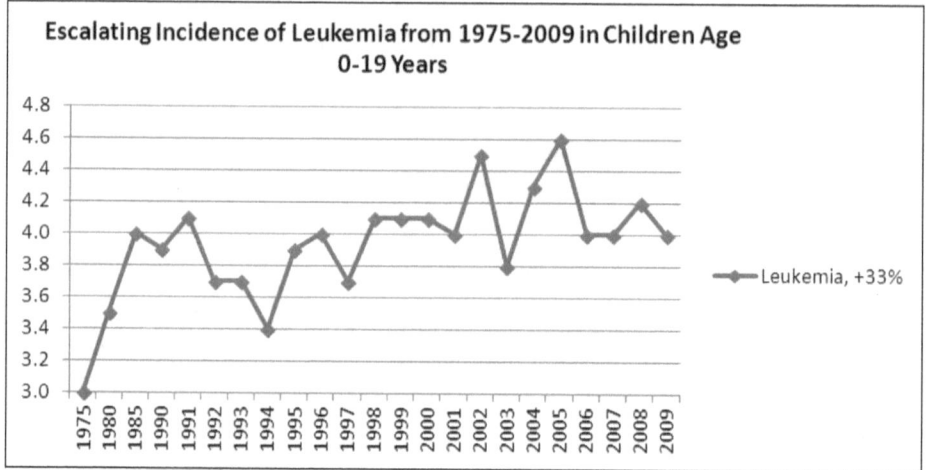

- Leukemias represents 31% of all cancers among children younger than 15 years of age, and 25% of cancer cases among those younger than 20. The relative contribution of leukemia to the total childhood cancer burden varies markedly with age, 17% in the first year of life, increasing to 46% for 2 and 3 year olds, and then decreasing to 9% for 19 year olds.
- The two major types of leukemia are acute lymphocytic leukemia (ALL), comprising nearly 75% and acute non-lymphocytic comprising 19%, of all leukemias.
- There is a sharp peak in the ALL incidence among 2-3 year olds, decreasing to 20 per million for 8-10 year olds.
- Leukemia rates are substantially higher for white than black children under 14 years, with rates of 46 versus 28 per million, respectively.
- The incidence of leukemia among children younger than 15 has shown a moderate increase in the past 20 years, primarily reflecting an increase in ALL incidence.

ACUTE LEUKEMIA

Incidence

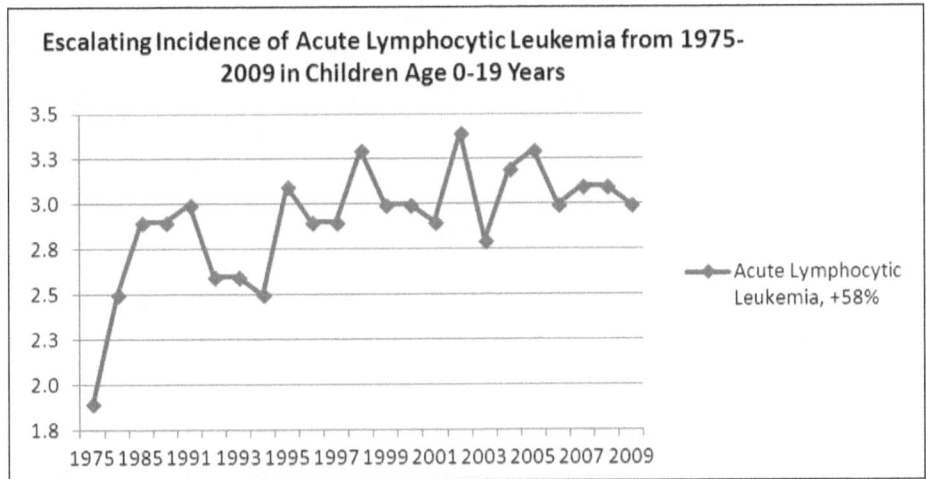

- Its incidence is higher in males than females, and in white than black children.
- Peak incidence age 2-5 years
- Prenatal and postnatal radiation exposure, including proximity of residence to nuclear power plants
- Genetic conditions such as Down and Bloom Syndrome
- With the exception of prenatal exposure to x-rays and specific genetic syndromes, little is known about its causes.
- Congenital genetic conditions such as neurofibroma and Li Fraumeni syndrome
- Radiation of scalp for treatment of tinea capitis (ringworm), neurofibromatosis, and Li-Fraumeni syndrome

LIVER CANCER

Incidence

- Primary neoplasms of the liver are rare in children, comprising only 1.1% of malignancies for children younger than 20 years of age. In the US, 100-150 children are diagnosed with liver cancer each year.
- Primary liver cancer is subdivided into the following histologic subtypes: hepatoblastoma comprises over two-thirds of the malignant

tumors of the liver in children and adolescents (79% <15 years of age; 66% <20 years of age) and hepatocellular carcinoma accounts for most of the remaining cases. Hepatoblastoma occurs primarily in children younger than 5 years of age while hepatocellular carcinoma occurs primarily after 10 years of age.
- The rate of hepatoblastoma was highest among infants with rates rapidly declining with increasing age. In contrast, the incidence of hepatocellular carcinoma increased as age increased.
- For those younger than 20 years of age, there was little change in liver cancer incidence during the 21-year period, with rates between 1.4 and 1.6 per million throughout the time period.
- The incidence of hepatoblastoma for children younger than 15 years of age increased during the 1975-95 period while the incidence of hepatocellular carcinoma decreased during the same period.

Survival

- Five-year survival rates for children with hepatoblastoma improved from 51% to 59% between 1976-84 and 1985-94. Survival rates were substantially lower for children and adolescents with hepatocellular carcinoma, with an improvement in 5-year survival rates from 31% for the years 1976-84 to 42% for the years 1985-94.

Risk factors

- The etiology of hepatoblastoma is as yet unknown but there are some tantalizing clues.

BONE CANCER

Incidence

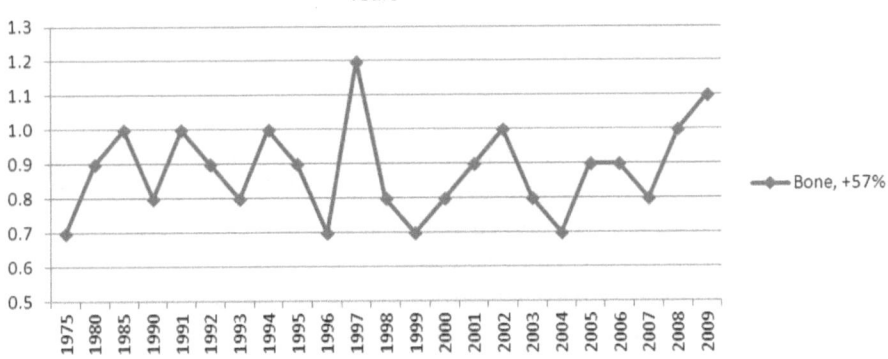

- Malignancies of the bone, with an average annual incidence rate of 8.7 per million children younger than 20 years of age, comprised about 6% of childhood cancer reported by SEER areas from 1975-95.
- In the US, 650-700 children and adolescents younger than 20 years of age are diagnosed with bone tumors each year of which approximately 400 are osteosarcoma and 200 are Ewing's sarcoma.
- The two types of malignant bone cancer that predominated in children were osteosarcomas and Ewing's sarcomas, about 56% and 34% of the malignant bone tumors, respectively.
- Osteosarcomas derive from primitive bone-forming mesenchymal stem cells and most often occur near the metaphyseal portions of the long bones. The Ewing's sarcomas are believed to be of neural crest origin and occur roughly evenly between the extremities and the central axis.
- For all bone cancer combined, a steady rise in incidence rates occurred with increasing age between ages 5 and 10, and a steeper rise began at age 11 until age 15 coinciding with the adolescent growth spurt. The peak incidence of bone cancer (19 per million) occurred at age 15, after which rates showed a decline.
- Rates did not differ much by sex among younger children, but males had higher incidence than females during adolescence.

- For osteosarcoma, black children had a higher overall rate than did white children. For Ewing's sarcoma the racial variation in rates was dramatic: white children had an approximate 6-fold higher incidence rate than black children.
- The most frequent site of bone cancer development was the long bones of the lower limbs for osteosarcomas and the central axis for Ewing's sarcomas.

Survival

- The 5-year relative survival for children with bone cancer improved from 49% in the period 1975-84, to 63% in the period 1985-94. The survival rates improved between the two time periods for both osteosarcoma and Ewing's sarcoma.
- Survival rates for osteosarcoma were higher than those for Ewing's sarcoma especially in the earlier time period.

Risk factors

- Although directed ionizing radiation exposure and a few genetic susceptibility syndromes are associated with increased risk of osteosarcoma, to date no factor has emerged to explain even a modest proportion of cases. Other than the important racial difference in incidence between black and white children, no environmental factor or other characteristic has yet been shown to be a strong risk factor for Ewing's sarcoma

RETINOBLASTOMA

Incidence

- Retinoblastoma accounted for approximately 11% of cancers developing in the first year of life, but for only 3% of the cancers developing among children younger than 15 years of age.
- In the US, approximately 300 children and adolescents younger than 20 years of age are diagnosed with retionblastomas each year.
- The vast majority of cases of retinoblastoma occur among young children, with almost two-thirds (63%) of all retinoblastomas occurring before the age of two years and 95% occurring before the age of five years.

- The incidence of bilateral tumors was strongly age dependent with 42% of the retinoblastomas occurring in children less than one year of age being bilateral compared to 21% of those among children aged one year, and only 9% among older children.
- Rates of retinoblastoma were essentially equal among males (3.7 per million) and females (3.8 per million), and among whites (3.7 per million) and blacks (4.0 per million).
- There was no substantial sustained change in retinoblastoma incidence during the 21-year period, 1975-95.

Survival

- Survival for children with retinoblastoma was favorable, with more than 93% alive at five years after diagnosis. Males and females had similar 5-year survival rates for the period 1976-94 (93-94%). Black children had slightly lower 5-year survival rates than white children (89% versus 94%).

Risk factors

- A retinoblastoma gene has been identified. Each child of a parent with familial bilateral retinoblastoma has a 50% risk of inheriting the retinoblastoma gene. Some patients develop the gene as the result of a new mutation (sporadic heritable retinoblastoma) and can pass the gene on to their children even though they did not inherit the gene from their parents. Children who inherit the retinoblastoma gene have a 90% risk of developing retinoblastoma. Genetic retinoblastomas are more likely to be bilateral and to occur during the first year of life. Little is know about non-genetic (sporadic) retinoblastomas.

SYMPATHEIC NERVOUS SYSTEM CANCER

Incidence

- In the US, approximately 700 children and adolescents younger than 20 years of age are diagnosed with tumors of the sympathetic nervous system each year, of which approximately 650 are neuroblastomas.
- Sympathetic nervous system tumors accounted for 7.8% of all cancers among children younger than 15 years of age.

- Over 97% of sympathetic nervous system tumors are neuroblastomas, embryonal malignancies of the sympathetic nervous system that occur almost exclusively in infants and very young children.
- Regardless of age, neuroblastomas most commonly occurred in the adrenal gland. Mediastinal tumors were more frequent in infants than in older children, while the opposite age pattern was observed for CNS tumors.
- The average age-adjusted annual incidence rate for all sympathetic nervous system cancers was 9.5 per million children.
- The occurrence of sympathetic nervous system malignancies was strongly age-dependent. For neuroblastomas alone, the incidence rate for both sexes combined during the second year of life (29 per million) was less than half that of infancy (64 per million).
- Neuroblastomas were by far the most common cancer of infancy, with an incidence rate almost double that of leukemia, the next most common malignancy that occurred during the first year of life.
- Sixteen percent of infant neuroblastomas were diagnosed during the first month following birth and 41% were diagnosed during the first 3 months of life.
- Over the 21-year observation period, there was little indication of an increase in the overall incidence of sympathetic nervous system malignancies. The estimated annual percent change in age-adjusted incidence rates was 0.4%.

Survival

- For children aged 1 to 4 years at diagnosis, 5-year survival rate improved from 35% during 1975-84 to 55% during 1985-94. Survival at 5 years from diagnosis was essentially unchanged over these time intervals among infants (83%) and children 5 years or older (40%).

Risk factors

- Relatively little is known about the etiology of sympathetic nervous system tumors. The young age at onset of most cases illustrates the need to investigate exposure events occurring before conception and during gestation.

CANCERS AND SARCOMAS

CANCERS

Incidence

- Among children, particularly before the adolescent years, carcinomas are very rare.
- In the US, approximately 1,050 children and adolescents younger than 20 years of age are diagnosed with carcinomas each year, of which approximately 350 are thyroid carcinomas and 300-350 are melanomas.
- All of the carcinomas combined comprised 9.2% of cancer in children younger than
- 20. The majority of the carcinomas were either thyroid carcinomas (35.5%) or melanomas (30.9%). Adrenocortical carcinomas (1.3%), nasopharyngeal carcinomas (4.5%), and other skin carcinomas (0.5%) combined for only a small proportion of the total, while other and unspecified carcinomas comprised 27.3%.
- The incidence rates for thyroid carcinoma were highest among the 15-19 year olds and much higher among females (24.4 per million) than males (4.7 per million).
- The incidence rates for malignant melanoma were highest among the 15-19 year olds and higher among females (16.5 per million) than males (10.0 per million).

Survival

- The 5-year survival rate was 99% for thyroid carcinomas. Males had a slightly lower survival rate than females.
- The 5-year survival rate was 91% for malignant melanoma. Females had a 93% survival rate compared to males with an 87% survival rate.

Risk factors

- The most well established risk factor for thyroid carcinoma is ionizing radiation exposure, from both environmental and therapeutic sources.
- The primary risk factors for melanoma are sun exposure and number of melanocytic and dysplastic nevi.

SARCOMAS

Incidence

- The soft tissue sarcomas of children and adolescents arise primarily from the connective tissues of the body, such as fibrous tissue, adipose tissue, and muscle tissue. The sarcomas that arise from bone are discussed separately in the bone tumor chapter.
- In the US, 850-900 children and adolescents younger than 20 years of age are diagnosed with soft tissue sarcomas each year, of which approximately 350 are rhabdomyosarcomas.
- The incidence of soft tissue sarcomas for children and adolescents younger than 20 years of age was 11.0 per million, representing 7.4% of cancer cases for this age group.
- Rhabdomyosarcoma was the most common soft tissue sarcoma among children 0-14 years, representing nearly 50% of soft tissue sarcomas for this age range with an incidence rate of 4.6 per million.
- There are two major types of rhabdomyosarcoma: embryonal (about 75% of rhabdomyosarcoma cases) and alveolar. These two subtypes tended to occur at different body sites and had different age patterns. The incidence of embryonal rhabdomyosarcoma was higher among children 0-4 years, while the incidence of alveolar rhabdomyosarcoma was similar throughout childhood.
- Other types of soft tissue sarcomas are rare and the incidence is higher in adolescents compared to younger children. Among these are the fibrosarcomas, malignant fibrous histiocytoma, synovial sarcoma, leiomyosarcoma, liposarcoma, and others.
- For infants, the most common soft tissue sarcoma was embryonal rhabdomyosarcoma. However, a distinctive set of other soft tissue sarcomas can develop in infants (e.g., infantile fibrosarcoma and malignant hemangiopericytoma). These tumors are different from the types of soft tissue sarcomas that arise in adolescents.
- Males had slightly higher incidence rates for soft tissue sarcomas than females for the period 1975-95.
- Black children had slightly higher incidence rates for soft tissue sarcomas than white children, with the largest difference observed among 15-19 year olds.
- The incidence of soft tissue sarcomas among those younger than 20 years of age has not changed much between 1975-79 (10.2 per million) and 1990-95 (11.3 per million).

Survival

- The overall 5-year survival rate for children with rhabdomyosarcoma was approximately 64% for cases diagnosed from 1985-94. Younger children had higher survival rates than older children and adolescents, and children with embryonal rhabdomyosarcoma had a more favorable prognosis than children with alveolar rhabdomyosarcoma.

Risk factors

- Congenital anomalies and genetic conditions are the only known risk factors for soft tissue sarcomas.

KNOWN CAUSES OF CHILDHOOD CANCERS*

Cancer	Risks
Lymphoid leukemia	Dental radiation Domestic pesticides Parental occupational carcinogens Genetic predisposition
Myeloid leukemia	Cancer drugs Genetic predisposition
Brain cancer	Radiation to the head Genetic predisposition
Thyroid cancer	Radiation to the head
Hodgkin's disease	Family history
Bone (osteosarcoma)	Radiation Cancer drugs Genetic predisposition
Ewing's sarcoma	Race, particularly white children
Neuroblastoma	None known
Retinoblastoma	None known
Kidney	Congenital
Muscle	Congenital
Liver	Genetic predisposition
Testicular	Undescended testicle

* Based in part on Pizzo and Poplack. *Principles and Practice of Pediatric Oncology 6th edition*. Philadelphia: Lippincott Williams & Wilkins, 2011.

AVOIDABLE CAUSES OF CANCER IN SCHOOLS*

"Schools may contain hidden and unexpected hazards, including cancer, and children spend as much time there ever day as does any workman in a factory or plant. Parents should check on the location of the school, to make sure that it is not near a chemical, mining, or smelting plant, or too close to busy highways and other sources of chemical emissions. The elementary school in Saugus, California, where about 3 ppm levels of the potent carcinogen vinyl chloride were found in classrooms in the summer of 1977, is a good case in point. The construction of the school building should also be examined to avoid the experience of several schools in Howell Township, New Jersey, in which friable asbestos-sprayed surfaces, such as soundproof ceilings, were found in 1976 to be liberating large quantities of asbestos fibers into the air.

"Laboratory courses should not expose students to harmful chemicals. Wood and metal shops should avoid the use of organic cleaning fluids and solvents containing benzene, carbon tetrachloride, or other carcinogens. Ventilation must be adequate. Chemistry laboratories and stockrooms should be completely cleared of all carcinogenic and other toxic chemicals, such as benzene. Some people question whether organic chemistry should be taught at all at the high school level. If it is, all chemicals used in classroom or laboratory work should be cleared by knowledgeable independent authority. Finally, the unsupervised use of toxic and carcinogenic pesticides by janitorial staff should be strictly banned."

---

* EPSTEIN, S.S. *The Politics of Cancer.* San Francisco: Sierra Club Books, 1978.

RISKS OF CANCER FROM PERSONAL CARE PRODUCTS

Why has the incidence of childhood cancers increased by about 40 percent over the past three decades? Could it have anything to do with the cancer causing (carcinogenic) ingredients in a wide range of personal care products which still crowd supermarket and other store shelves?

Most of us would like to believe that any such products, especially those marketed for infants and children, must be safe or they would never be sold. Surely, the Food and Drug Administration (FDA), the responsible agency of government, besides the industry concerned, must be looking out for the health of our most vulnerable citizens. Right? Wrong!

In fact, babies are about 100 times more sensitive to carcinogens than adults. Infants and young children have immature liver enzymes, which give them only limited ability to detoxify the carcinogens and other toxic ingredients in products which are applied to their skin. Also, as children's cells divide much more rapidly than those of adults, they are much more sensitive to carcinogens, and more vulnerable to developing cancer later in their lives.

Added to all of that is the fact that the ingredients in the products we apply to the skin of our infants and children are readily absorbed into their bodies. Also, they are retained for much longer than any chemicals absorbed from food or from the air.

So, as detailed in my 2010 *Healthy Beauty* book[*], there is every reason why we should be highly cautious about the personal care products that we buy for our children.

---

[*]   Co-authored by R. Fitzgerald.

INGREDIENT	TOXIC EFFECT(S)[*]
Benzyl alcohol	Allergen
Cetearaths	Contaminated with the carcinogens ethylene oxide and dioxane
Diazolidinyl Urea	Precursor of the carcinogen formaldehyde
DMDM Hydantoin	Precursor of the carcinogen formaldehyde
EDTA	Hormone disrupter and penetration enhancer
FD&C Red 40	Carcinogen
Lanolin	Allergen
Laureths	Contaminated with the carcinogens ethylene oxide and dioxane
Parabens	Hormone disruptors
Polyethylene glycol (PEG)	Contaminated with the carcinogens ethylene oxide and dioxane
Polysorbates	Contaminated with the carcinogens ethylene oxide and dioxane
Quaternium-15	Precursor of the carcinogen formaldehyde
Sodium lauryl sulfate	Penetration enhancer
Talc (talcum powder)	Carcinogen and lung irritant
Triethanolamine (TEA)	Precursor of the carcinogen nitrosamine

Worse still, that threat begins even before birth. Once a pregnant woman absorbs ingredients from the cosmetics and personal care products that she uses, they penetrate through her skin to varying degrees. They then reach the fetus through the approximately 300 quarts of blood pumped daily between the placenta and fetus.

Studies on umbilical and blood cord samples have identified antibacterial ingredients, such as triclosan, often added to deodorants, toothpaste, and cosmetics. Based on rodent tests, triclosan has also been shown to have toxic effects on liver enzymes.

These umbilical and blood cord studies have also identified hormonal ingredients such as phthalates, which are used as solvents in perfumes, lotions and other cosmetics.

Of major concern, exposure to some phthalates has been shown to disturb the hormonal and sexual development of boys, even at relatively low levels.

University of Liverpool toxico-pathologist Dr. Vyvyan Howard describes the significance of these findings for the fetal stage of life, warning, "Changes

---

[*] EPSTEIN, S.S and FITZGERALD, R. *Healthy Beauty*, BenBella Books, 2009.

occur at exposure levels thousands of times lower than the safety limits that were set a few years ago.

"New studies show that many bulk chemicals that we thought were safe are actually biologically active and disrupt human systems. They don't work by having an acute toxicity effect. They work by hijacking development in the uterus. These chemicals can disrupt important cell signaling functions in the developing body," Dr. Howard says.

Once a child is born, this susceptibility to hormonal ingredients in cosmetics and personal care products persists. One of the biggest culprits, incriminated for disrupting sex hormones in boys, is Bisphenol-A (BPA). This is a plasticizer which mimics the effects of the hormone estrogen, and is a common ingredient in cosmetics and personal care products.

Males, both human and rodent, have been shown to be more sensitive to these hormonal ingredients than females. Male rodents exposed to BPA and other related ingredients have developed testicular atrophy, undescended or absent testes, infertility, an absent or malformed prostate and seminal vesicles, and also cancer. Decreased sperm production and a decrease in the distance between the anus and genitals in infant boys have also been documented over the past few decades.

Women are also adversely affected by exposure to BPA. Tests on rodents, as reported in the journal "Reproductive Toxicology" and elsewhere, have revealed that BPA may be responsible for reproductive disorders later in life, decades after their exposure to the chemical in the womb or as infants.

We know that babies being born today have elevated levels of hormonal phthalates in their bodies. A 2008 study in the journal "Pediatrics" confirmed this by testing the urine of babies who had just been shampooed, lotioned or powdered with brand-name baby products. Similar results came from studies done by the *U.S. Centers for Disease Control and Prevention*.

Based on this disturbing data, in 2008 Health Canada ruled that BPA is a toxic ingredient. However, no such warning has yet come from the U.S. Food and Drug Administration.

Besides toxic hormonal effects, there are other dangers posed by products marketed for infants and children. Here are a few examples:

- Allergens such as benzyl alcohol and lanolin commonly appear.
- Carcinogens such as formaldehyde appears when product ingredients DMDM Hydantoin and Quaternium-15 break down
- Carcinogens found in shampoos and conditioners include the laureths as well as dioxane and ethylene oxide.

- Penetration enhancer ingredients that drive other ingredients deeper through the skin into the body are common. These include sodium lauryl sulfate and EDTA.

Nevertheless, the mainstream cosmetics industry continues to insist that none of their products are harmful, as their levels of toxic ingredients are claimed to be too low to pose any dangers.

Even if this were true, it's a flawed argument. It ignores how infants and children are subjected to multiple assaults of multiple toxic ingredients from a wide range of personal care products applied to their skin each day.

Importantly, we must consider the additive and multiplistic effects of all these chemicals interacting together.

Safe skin products for infants and children are now increasingly available on store shelves for responsible parents. These include USDA certified organic products. These leading products are detailed in the 2009 *Toxic Beauty* book.

Additionally, the Environmental Working Group maintains a database at www.cosmeticsdatabase.com/special/parentsguide/ which provides information on toxic ingredients in children's products, and on safer products.

Under the explicit provisions of the 1938 Federal Food, Drug and Cosmetic Act, it is anticipated that Dr. Margaret Hamburg, the newly appointed FDA Commissioner and inspiring public health advocate, will prohibit the sale of toxic personal care products for children.

UNIQUE CANCER RISKS FROM COSMETICS AND PERSONAL CARE PRODUCTS

Mainstream cosmetics and personal care products (CPCPs) are the single most important, yet generally unrecognized, class of avoidable carcinogenic exposures for overwhelming majority of children, besides adults, in the U.S. and other major industrialized nations. The reason for these unique risks reflects a complex of individual and interactive factors. As warned by Senator Edward Kennedy in 1997 in Senate hearings on the FDA Reform Bill, "The cosmetic industry has borrowed a page from the playbook of the tobacco industry by putting profits ahead of public health."

Interaction between Different Carcinogenic Ingredients

Serious as is the absorption of any single carcinogenic ingredient, particularly from large areas of skin, this is relatively trivial compared to the lifetime absorption of a variety of carcinogenic ingredients, totaling some 70, in multiple CPCPs. While the effects of numerous carcinogens are minimally additive, there is limited evidence that they are likely to be multiplicative or synergistic.

Prolonged Duration of Exposure

Exposure to carcinogenic CPCP ingredients is cumulative over childhood from multiple different products. In fact, exposure precedes birth from maternal skin absorption at the earliest stages of pregnancy. Furthermore, apart from wash-off products, most others are applied to and remain on the skin for prolonged periods of time.

High Permeability of Skin

Skin is a highly porous membrane, approximately one-twentieth of an inch think. As such, the skin is permeable to carcinogenic and other toxic ingredients, especially following prolonged exposure. A 1989 study showed that 13 percent of the carcinogenic preservative butylated hydroxytoluene (BHT) and 50 percent of the carcinogenic pesticide DDT, which often contaminate the common non-carcinogenic ingredient lanolin, are rapidly absorbed through human skin. Even more disturbing is evidence that the permeability of skin to carcinogens may be greater than that of the intestines. In evidence presented at 1978 Congressional hearings, the absorption of nitrosodiethanolamine (NDELA) formed by the nitrosation of DEA, is over 100 times greater from the skin than by mouth. This is particularly important as consumption of the closely related carcinogen, diethylnitrosamine, in nitrite-preserved bacon has been associated with up to 4—and 7-fold increased risks of childhood brain cancer and leukemia, respectively.

Carcinogenic Ingredients In Cosmetics and Personal Care Products

Personal care products, manufactured and marketed by most mainstream and multilevel marking industries and companies, are still veritable "witches brews" of multiple carcinogenic ingredients and contaminants, besides unrelated toxics. However, only minimal or no such information is disclosed to the public.

Apart from those few products, notably talc, which themselves are carcinogens, there are 3 major classes of carcinogenic ingredients. The first includes over 40 ingredients that are carcinogenic themselves, and known as "frank" carcinogens, some of which also induce genetic damage. The second are 30 "hidden" carcinogens, which are precursors of carcinogens. The third are 7 carcinogenic ingredients which also induce genetic damage, and known as "genotoxic" carcinogens (Epstein, S.S., Unreasonable Risk, Environment Toxicology, Inc. 2005).

EVIDENCE ON CANCER RISKS FROM COSMETICS AND PERSONAL CARE PRODUCTS

What is the source of evidence on the carcinogenicity of ingredients in cosmetics and personal care products (CPCPs), and just how reliable is this? Evidence on their carcinogenicity is detailed in numerous sources. These include: a series of 83 International Agency for Research on Cancer (IARC) monographs published since 1972, each detailing different classes of industrial and other chemicals; some 600 National Institutes of Health Technical Report Series on individual carcinogens now published by the Federal National toxicology Program (NTP), based on rodent tests; the NTP's supposedly annual Report on carcinogens, initiated in 1978, although only 10 have since been published, summarizing evidence on a limited number of carcinogens identified in animal tests or human studies; numerous articles in scientific publications that are virtually inaccessible or incomprehensible to the general public, which report the results of animal test and human epidemiological studies; and the compilation, analysis and interpretation of all existing evidence in referenced publications.

Additional sources of information on the carcinogenicity of PCP ingredients include: the 1980 Science Action Coalition's Consumer's Guide to Cosmetics; the author's books including the 1995 Safe Shopper's Bible, the 1998 Breast Cancer Prevention Program, the 1998 The Politics of Cancer Revisited, the 2009 Healthy Beauty, and a wide range of information from the Cancer Prevention Coalition. This includes its extensive and user-friendly website *www.preventcancer.com*, with some 270 press releases, many dealing with CPCPs. Finally, evidence on the carcinogenicity of CPCP ingredients and contaminants is now admitted, although trivializing so, in the Cosmetic

Ingredient Review, published annually by the Cosmetic, Toiletry and Fragrance Association.

It should be emphasized that testing for carcinogenicity, besides related toxicity of CPCPs, must be conducted on the products' ingredients and contaminants, rather than on the whole products themselves. Tests on the latter would be too insensitive to detect the carcinogenic effects of individual ingredients and contaminants, let alone determine which are responsible. This is especially critical in view of the relatively low concentrations of carcinogenic ingredient in any product. An additional concern is the small number of rodents used in standard test protocols. Thus, statements proclaiming "Not Tested On Animals" usually relate to the whole product, generally irritation, or allergy tests in rabbits or guinea pigs, rather than ingredients in the product.

TOXIC INGREDIENTS IN INFANTS' AND CHILDREN'S PRODUCTS

CHEMICAL NAME	EXPOSUSRE AND TOXIC EFFECTS	CURRENT STATUS NTP*
Acesulfame potassium	<ul><li>Widely used as a component of Splenda sweetener blends, and in sweetened products such as "lite" fruit juices, fruit drinks, ice creams, flavored water and sports drinks</li><li>Inadequate long-term animal testing</li><li>Tests carried out to date do not give reasonable assurance that acesulfame potassium is "safe"</li><li>Two-year toxicity/carcinogenicity studies in rats and mice</li></ul>	In review/pending
Bisphenol A	<ul><li>There is a widespread exposure to low doses of Bisphenol A</li><li>Developmental reproductive effects</li></ul>	Selected

---

* National Toxicology Program. 12th Report on Carcinogens. 2012.

CHEMICAL NAME	EXPOSUSRE AND TOXIC EFFECTS	CURRENT STATUS NTP
Di (2-ethylhexyl) phthalate (DEHP)	• Long-term risks associated with medical exposures of infants to DEHP have not been clearly elucidated significant knowledge gaps on the toxicokinetics and effects in fetal and neonatal primates of intravenous DEHP exposure • Further studies will better define risks and benefits of utilizing non-DEHP-containing products	In review/pending
2-Methoxy-4-nitroaniline	• Used in dyeing textiles and toy enamels • Chronic toxicity, developmental, reproductive • Toxicological characterization including chronic toxicity and carcinogenicity studies	Selected
Triclosan	• Widespread use in consumer products • Frequent and long-term exposure for all age groups • Lack of adequate toxicity data for dermal exposures • Carcinogenicity studies via dermal administration	In review/pending
Diacetyl (artificial butter flavoring)	• Several outbreaks of fatal lung disease have been documented among workers exposed to the vapors of butter flavoring in the manufacture of popcorn, the most prominent chemical exposures being from diacetyl and acetonin • The potency and severity of diacetyl has been demonstrated by short-term laboratory tests. • Toxicity, carcinogenicity by inhalation	Selected

CANCER RISKS FROM PERSONAL CARE PRODUCTS*

Talcum Powder (Johnson & Johnson. Inc.)

Labeled Toxic Ingredient:
Talc: Carcinogenic and a risk factor for ovarian cancer; lung irritant.

Note: Substantive evidence of causal relation to ovarian cancer.

Safer Alternative:
Corn Starch—(Johnson & Johnson, Inc.)

Cover Girl Replenishing Natural Finish Make-Up (Foundation)

Labeled Toxic Ingredients:
BHA: Carcinogenic; Talc: Carcinogenic; Titanium Dioxide: Carcinogenic; Triethanolamine
(TEA): interacts with nitrites to form carcinogenic nitrosamines; Lanolin: often contaminated with DDT and other carcinogenic pesticides.

Crest Tartar Control Toothpaste (Procter & Gamble. Inc.)

Labeled Toxic Ingredients:
FD&C BLUE #1: Carcinogenic.
Saccharin: Carcinogenic.
Fluoride: Possibly carcinogenic.

---

* EPSTEIN, S.S. *The Politics of Cancer, Revisited.* East Ridge Press, 1998.

Safer Alternative:
Tom's of Maine Natural Non-Fluoride Toothpaste

Alberto V05 Conditioner (Essence of Neutral Henna) (Alberto-Culver USA, Inc.)

Labeled Toxic Ingredients:
Formaldehyde: Carcinogenic; Polysorbate 80: can be contaminated with the carcinogen 1,4-dioxane; FD&C Red #4: Carcinogenic.

Clairol Nice 'n Easy (Permanent Haircolor) (Clairol, Inc.)

Labeled Toxic Ingredients:
Quaternium-15: Formaldehyde releaser, Carcinogenic; Diethanolamine (DEA): interacts with nitrites to form a carcinogenic nitrosamine; Phenylendiamines: includes carcinogens and other ingredients inadequately tested for carcinogenicity. Note: Substantive evidence of causal relation to lymphoma, multiple myeloma, and other cancers.

CANCER RISKS FROM HOUSEHOLD PRODUCTS*

AJAX Cleanser (Colgate-Palmolive. Inc.)

Unlabeled Carcinogenic Ingredients:
Crystalline Silica: Carcinogenic; eye, skin and lung irritant.
Washing Soda:Caustic.
NOTE: Carcinogenicity of silica is stated in 1994 Material Safety and Data Sheet (MSDS).

Safer Alternative:
Comet Cleanser (Procter & Gamble, Inc.)

Zud Heavy Duty Cleanser (Reckitt & Colman. Inc.)

Unlabeled Carcinogenic Ingredient:
Crystalline Silica: Carcinogenic; eye, skin and lung irritant. (Carcinogenicity is denied in MSDS.)

Safer Alternative:
Comet Cleanser (Procter & Gamble, Inc.)

---

* EPSTEIN, S.S. *The Politics of Cancer, Revisited.* East Ridge Press, 1998.

Lysol Disinfectant Spray (Reckitt & Colman. Inc.)

Labeled or Unlabeled Carcinogenic Ingredient:
Orthophenylphenol (OPP): Carcinogenic; irritant. (Carcinogenicity is denied in MSDS.)

Safer Alternative:
Airwick Stick Up (Reckitt & Colman, Inc.)

Zodiac Cat & Dog Flea Collar (Sandoz Agro. Inc).

Labeled Carcinogenic Ingredient
Propoxur: Carcinogenic; neurotoxic.

Safer Alternative:
Trader Joe's Herbal Flea Collar for cats or dogs

Ortho Weed-B-Gon Lawn Weed Killer (Monsanto Co.)

Labeled Carcinogenic Ingredient
Sodium 2,4-Dichlorophenoxyacetate (2,4-D): Carcinogenic with evidence of casual relation to lymphoma, soft tissue sarcoma and other cancers; neurotoxic; reproductive toxin.NOTE: Substantive evidence of causation to lymphoma, soft tissue sarcoma, and other cancers.

Safer Alternative:
Organic pesticides.

CANCER RISKS FROM FOOD*

Beef Frankfurters

Unlabeled Toxic Ingredients
Benzene hexachloride: Carcinogenic.
Dacthal: Carcinogenic (can be contaminated with dioxin); irritant; strong sensitizer.
Dieldrin, Carcinogenic; xenoestrogen.
DDT: Carcinogenic; xenoestrogen.
Heptachlor: Carcinogenic; neurotoxic; reproductive toxin; xenoestrogen.
Hexachlorobenzene: Carcinogenic; neurotoxic; teratogenic.
Lindane: Carcinogenic; neurotoxic; damage to blood forming cells.
Hormones: Carcinogenic and feminizing.
Antibiotics: Some are carcinogenic (eg. sulfamethazine).

Note: substantive evidence of causal relation to childhood cancer

Labeled Ingredient
Nitrite: Interacts with meat amines to form carcinogenic nitrosamines which are a major risk factor for childhood cancers.

Safer Alternative:
Nitrite-Free Organic hot dogs or tofu franks.

---

* EPSTEIN, S.S. *The Politics of Cancer, Revisited*. East Ridge Press, 1998.

Whole Milk—(eg. Borden or Lucerne)

Unlabeled Toxic Ingredients
DDT: Carcinogenic; xenoestrogen.
Dieldrin: Carcinogenic; xenoestrogen.
Heptachlor: Carcinogenic; neurotoxic; reproductive toxin; xenoestrogen.
Hexachlorobenzene: Carcinogenic; neurotoxic; reproductive toxin.
Antibiotics: Some are carcinogenic, cause allergies and drug resistance.
Recombinant Bovine Growth Hormone (rBGH) and IGF-1.

Note: Substantive evidence of breast, colon and prostate cancer promotion.

Safer Alternative:
rBGH-free Organic skim milk

HOW TO AVOID CHILDHOOD CANCER AND HORMONAL RISKS

On September 10, 1997, at Senate hearings on the FDA Reform Bill, Senator Kennedy warned that "The cosmetics industry has borrowed a page from the playbook of the tobacco industry by putting profits ahead of public health." However, this warning remains recklessly ignored by the Food and Drug Administration (FDA), and unknown by the general public.

Conventional personal care products, besides cosmetics, still contain a wide range of toxic ingredients that pose risks of cancer, hormonal abnormalities, and allergies.

From 1975 to 2008, the overall incidence of childhood cancer under the age of 18, has increased by 32%, while mortality decreased by 55%. As warned in the author's 2009 *Healthy Beauty* book, babies and young children are up to 100 times more sensitive than adults to causes of cancer, known as carcinogens. Of additional concern is the increasing evidence of toxic hormonal effects, known as gender bending, in infants and young children. These include premature breast development in young girls and genital abnormalities in baby boys.

Scandously, all these risks still remain unknown by the public, and ignored by the Food and Drug Administration (FDA). However, they are now avoidable as safe organic products certified by the U.S. Department of Agriculture (USDA), are readily available. These include: Aubrey Organics

Baby and Kids Soaps, Dr. Bronner's Bath Soaps, and organic cornstarch baby powder.

On December 3, 2009, reflecting on these concerns, Senator John Kerry and Congressman Jim Moran introduced a joint bill, the Endocrine Disruption Act of 2009, designed to enable governmental action "to explore linkages between hormone disrupting chemicals in the environment and everyday goods and the dramatic increase of . . . . breast, prostate and other cancers. From laundry detergent to pesticides, and from fire retardant clothing to plastic baby bottles, these products are potential vehicles for human exposure to endocrine disruptive chemicals whose long term health effects are still unknown." These concerns were further supported by Dr. Aydin and colleagues, who published a January 2011 article in the *Journal of the National Cancer Institute* reporting on the relation of mobile phone use and brain cancer in children and adolescents.

SURVIVAL*

- The prognosis for infants with a particular cancer is often worse than in children of older ages.
- Overall 5-year survival rates for adolescents with cancer has improved from 69% to 77% over recent decades.
- For some types of cancer (Hodgkin's disease, germ cell tumors, thyroid cancer, and melanoma), 5-year survival rates are 90%.
- For other cancer types (e.g., osteosarcoma, Ewing's sarcoma, ALL, and AML) survival rates for adolescents remain less than 60%.
- Over 80% of children diagnosed with neuroblastoma during infancy are alive 5 years following diagnosis. In contrast, for children diagnosed with neuroblastoma at age 1 year or older, the 5-year relative survival is about 45%.
- The 5-year survival rate was 99% for thyroid carcinomas. Males had a slightly lower survival rate than females.
- The 5-year survival rate was 91% for malignant melanoma. Females had a 93% survival rate compared to males with an 87% survival rate.

---

* National Cancer Institute (NCI) SEER Pediatric Monograph, 1995.

CARCINOGENIC PESTICIDES*

Acifluorfen	DDT	Propargite**
Acrylonitrile	Daminozide	Propazine
Alachlor	Unsymmetrical 1,1-dimethylhydrazine	Propoxur
Aldrin	Dichloroethyl ether	Trichloroethene
Amitrole	1,2-dichloropropane	Safrole
Ethylene thiourea	Dichloropropene	Dihydrosafrole
B naphthylamine	Dichlorvos	Simazine**
Aramite	Dicofol**	Tetrachlorvinphos (TCVP)
Arsenic	4-chloroaniline	Trifluralin**
Arsenic trioxide	Dihydrosafrole	Toxaphene
Sodium arsenate (II)	Dimethylnitrosamine	2,4,6-Trichlorophenol
Atrazine	Epichlorohydrin	2,7-dichlorodibenzo-p-dioxin
Auramine	N-nitrosodipropylamine	DBCP
Azobenzene	Ethylfulralin	Naphtha
Benzene	Ethylene dibromide	Procymidone
Benzene hexachloride	Ethylene dichloride	
N-nitrosomethyl-n-butylamine	Ethylene oxide	
Cadmium chloride	N-nitrosodimethylamine	
Cadmium oxide	Folpet	

---

* Briggs, Shirley A. Basic Guide to Pesticides: Their Characteristics and Hazards. Rachel Carson Council. 1992.

Cadmium sulfate	Formaldehyde	
Captafol	1,4-dioxane	
Captan	Heptachlor	
Nitrosocarbaryl	Hexachlorobenzene	
Carbon tetrachloride	Dipropylnitrosamine	
CDEC	Isoxaben	
Chloranil	Lindane	
Chlordane	Malaoxon	
Chlordecone	Mercuric chloride	
Chlordimeform	Metam sodium**	
4-chloro-o-toluidine	Methylene chloride	
N-formyl-chloro-o-toluidine	Methyl bromide**	
Chlorobenzilate	Mirex	
Chloroform	Monuron	
TCDD	N-nitrosonornicotine	
Chlorothalonil**	Perchloroethylene	
Creosote (coal tar)	PCBs	
Melamine	Pentachlorophenol	
2,4-D	Hexachlorodibenzo-p-dioxin	

** Agricultural pesticide

THE PRESIDENT'S CANCER PANEL WARNS OF ENVIRONMENTAL RISKS OF CANCER, 2008-2009 REPORT

Children Are At Special Risk for Cancer Due To Environmental Contaminants and Should Be Protected

"Opportunities for eliminating or minimizing cancer-causing and cancer-promoting environmental exposures must be acted upon to protect all Americans, but especially children. They are at special risk due to their smaller body mass and rapid physical development, both of which magnify their vulnerability to known or suspected carcinogens, including radiation. Numerous environmental contaminants can cross the placental barrier; to a disturbing extent, babies are born "pre-polluted." Children also can be harmed by genetic or other damage resulting from environmental exposures sustained by the mother (and in some cases, the father). There is a critical lack of knowledge and appreciation of environmental threats to children's health and a severe shortage of researchers and clinicians trained in children's environmental health."

The Special Vulnerabilities of Children

"Infants, children, and adolescents comprise 40 percent of the world's population. In crucial respects (e.g., ability to control their environment, ability to care for and defend themselves), they are the most vulnerable group. Mortality from childhood cancers has dropped dramatically since

1975 due to vastly improved treatments that have resulted from high levels of participation by children in cancer treatment clinical trials. Yet over the same period (1975-2008), cancer incidence in U.S. children under 20 years of age increased." Tests of umbilical cord blood found traces of nearly 300 pollutants in newborns' bodies, such as chemicals used in fast-food packaging, flame retardants present in household dust, and pesticides.

PARENTAL OCCUPATIONAL EXPOSURES POSE UNRECOGNIZED CANCER RISKS TO THEIR CHILDREN IN DEFIANCE OF THE FAMILY PROTECTION ACT*

Because of repeated reports of contamination of workers' homes, the Workers Family Protection Act, was introduced in 1991 in the U.S. Senate and the House of Representatives. In 1992, the U.S. Congress passed the Workers' Family Protection Act. This required the National Institute for Occupational Safety and Health (NIOSH) to conduct a study to "evaluate contamination of workers' homes with hazardous chemicals and substances (including infectious agents) . . . transported from their workplaces." NIOSH found that contamination of workers' homes was an extensive problem. Other incidents had also been reported by 36 U.S. states. These incidents resulted in a wide range of toxic effects and death among workers' families, particularly their children.

As required by the 1992 Act, NIOSH conducted a study on workers' home contamination in cooperation with the Secretary of Labor, the Administrator of the Environmental Protection Agency (EPA), the Administrator for the Agency for Toxic Substances and Disease Registry,

---

* Based on *Report to Congress on Worker's Home Contamination Study Conducted under the Worker's Family Protection Act*. September 1995.

and other appropriate Federal Government agencies. The study was based on two major concerns: 1) past incidents of home contamination as reported in the literature and in the records of NIOSH, the Occupational Safety and Health Administration (OSHA), the States, and other governmental agencies, including the Department of Energy (DOE) and the EPA; and 2) an evaluation of current statutory, regulatory, and voluntary industrial hygiene or other measures used by small, medium, and large employers to prevent or remediate home contamination.

The Act also directed NIOSH to report existing research and case histories conducted on incidents of employee transported contaminant releases, including:

- The health effects if any of the resulting exposure on workers and their families;
- Methods for differentiating exposure health effects and relative risks associate with specific agents from other sources of exposure inside and outside the home;
- The effectiveness of workplace housekeeping practices and personal protective equipment in preventing home contamination;
- The effectiveness of normal house cleaning and laundry procedures for decontaminating workers' homes and personal clothing; and
- Indoor air quality, as the research concerning such pertains to the fate of chemicals transported from a workplace into the home environment.

The Act also cited "Current knowledge on the causes of childhood brain cancer." This was ascribed to therapeutic radiation to the head, and congenital genetic conditions such as neurofibroma and the Li Fraumeni syndrome. The Act further cited "Current Knowledge" on the causes of congenital kidney cancer (Wilm's tumor), with reference to its higher incidence in whites than blacks.

The report further included: a survey of reported health effects, information on sources and levels of contamination; preventive measures; decontamination procedures; a review of Federal and State laws; and responses of agencies and industry to incidents involving contamination of workers' homes.

Health Effects of Workers' Home Contamination

Workers can inadvertently carry hazardous materials home from work on their clothes, skin, hair, tools, and in their vehicles. As a result, families of these workers, particularly their children, had been exposed to hazardous substances and have developed various health effects. Health effects have also occurred when the home and the workplace are not distinct—such as on farms or in homes that involve cottage industries. For some contaminants, there are other potential sources of home contamination such as air and water pollution and deteriorating lead paint in the home.

Little is still known of the full range of health effects or the extent to which they occur as a result of workers' home contamination. There are no information systems to enable tracking of illnesses and health conditions resulting from these circumstances. Many of the health effects among workers' family members described below. These were first recognized because of their uniqueness their clear relationship to workplace contaminants, or their serious nature.

- **Chronic beryllium disease**
  This potentially fatal lung disease has occurred in families of workers exposed to beryllium in the nuclear and aviation industries and workplaces involved in the production of beryllium and fluorescent lights and gyroscopes.
- **Asbestosis and mesothelioma**
  Fatal lung diseases have occurred among family members of workers engaged in the manufacture of many products containing asbestos, including thermal insulation materials, asbestos cement, automobile mufflers, shingles, textiles, gas masks, floor tiles, boilers, ovens, and brakeshoes and other friction products for automobiles. Families have also been exposed to asbestos when workers were engaged in mining, shipbuilding, insulation (e.g. pipe laggers and railway workers), maintenance and repair of boilers and vehicles, and asbestos removal operations.
- **Lead poisoning, neurological effects, and mental retardation**
  These health effects have occurred in children of workers engaged in mining, smelting, construction, manufacturing (pottery, ceramics, stained glass, ceramic tiles, electrical components, bullets, and lead batteries), repair and reclamation of lead batteries, repair of radiators, recovery of gold and silver, work on firing ranges, and welding, painting, and splicing of cables.
- **Deaths and neurological effects from pesticides**
  Farm families and families of other workers exposed to pesticides have suffered these serious effects.

- **Chemical burns from caustic substances**
  Chemical burns of the mouth and esophagus and fatalities from ingesting caustic substances have occurred in farm families when hazardous substances were improperly used and stored on farms.
- **Chloracne and other effects from chlorinated hydrocarbons**
  Family members have been exposed when these substances were transported home on clothing of workers manufacturing or using these compounds in the production of insulated wire, plastic products, ion exchange resins, and textiles. Family members have been similarly exposed when workers' clothes became contaminated during marine electrical work, transformer maintenance, municipal sewage treatment, rail transportation, wood treatment, and application of herbicides.
- **Neurological effects from mercury**
  Family members have developed various neurological effects as a result of being exposed to mercury carried home on clothing of workers engaged in mining, thermometer manufacture, and cottage-industry gold extraction.
- **Abnormal development from estrogenic substances**
  Enlarged breasts have occurred in boys and girls and premature menstruation has occurred in girls from estrogenic substances brought home on contaminated clothing of pharmaceutical and farm workers.
- **Asthmatic and allergic reactions from dusts**
  Farm families and others have suffered asthmatic and other allergic effects from animal allergens, mushrooms, gain dust, and platinum salts.
- **Liver angiosarcoma from arsenic**
  Families of workers engaged in mining, smelting, and wood treatment have been exposed to arsenic from contaminated skin and clothing; one child developed liver angiosarcoma.
- **Dermatitis from fibrous glass**
  Family members have developed dermatitis when their clothing was contaminated with fibrous glass during laundering of insulation workers' clothing
- **Epilepsy from chemical exposure**
  A child experienced epileptic seizures following ingestion of explosive compounds brought home on the clothing of a worker engaged in their manufacture.

- **Diseases from infectious agents**
  Family members have contracted infectious diseases, such as scabies and Q fever, from agents brought home on contaminated clothing and skin of workers engaged in agriculture, hospital, and laboratory work. As intended by Congress, infectious agents are included as hazardous substances to the extent that they can be brought home on a worker's skin or clothing.

Measures for Preventing Home Contamination

Preventive measures that were found to be effective when used in the workplace include:

- Reducing exposures in the workplace;
- Changing clothes before going home and leaving the soiled clothing at work to be laundered by the employer;
- Storing street clothes in separate areas of the workplace to prevent their contamination;
- Showering before leaving work; and
- Prohibiting removal of toxic substances or contaminated items from the workplace

Preventive measures that have been used successfully at home include:

- Separating work areas of cottage industries from living areas;
- Properly storing and disposing of toxic substances on farms and in cottage industries;
- Preventing family members from visiting the workplace;
- Laundering contaminated clothing separately from family laundry when it is necessary to launder contaminated clothing at home; and
- Informing workers of the risk to family members and of preventive measures.

Other preventive measures that need to be used include:

- Educating physicians and other health professionals to inquire about potential work-related causes of disease;
- Developing surveillance programs to track health effects that could be related to home contamination; and
- Educating children, parents, and teachers about the effects of toxic substances.

Recommendations for Research and Education

- The prevalence of health effects of contaminants transported from the workplace should be determined. One possible approach would be to conduct surveys among occupational and environmental medicine health care providers and clinics.
- The employment practices and controls that work best in preventing the transport of contaminants from the workplace to the home should be identified.
- Educational programs to prevent home contamination should be developed for employers, workers, children, teachers, and parents, physicians, and other health professionals.
- The special needs and problems of individuals who work in home or cottage industries need to be identified.

Conclusions

- Workers' home contamination may pose a serious public health problem. Health effects and deaths from contaminants brought home from the workplace have been reported in 28 countries and 36 States.
- The extent to which these health effects occur is not fully known as there are no effective information systems to tract them, and physicians do not always recognize the relationship between toxic occupational exposures and various common toxic effects.
- About half of the reports of health effects from home contamination are less than 10 years old. The literature on the health effects involved approximately 30 different substances or agents. The potential exists for many of the thousands of other chemicals used in commerce to be transported to workers' homes or to be sued in home-centered businesses.
- Health effects and deaths from contaminants brought home from the workplace are preventable using known effective measures. Educational programs are needed to promote their use.
- Normal house cleaning and laundry practices are often inadequate form decontaminating workers' homes and clothing and can increase the hazard to the person performing the tasks and others in the household.

- Only two Federal laws have had elements that directly address workers' home contamination. However, other laws provide agencies with certain mechanisms for responding to, or preventing workers' home contamination. Operating under existing laws the Centers for Disease Control (including NIOSH) and the National Center for Environmental Health have also responded to incidents of workers' home contamination, and made recommendations to prevent such incidents, and conducted relevant research.

THE PRESIDENT'S CANCER PANEL WARNS OF HORMONAL RISKS OF BISPHENOL-A

Bisphenol-A is widely used as a plasticizer in polycarbonate baby bottles, besides adult personal care and cosmetic products, food can linings, microwave oven dishes, dental sealants, and also medical devices. Other recently recognized major sources are cash register and credit-card receipts, which are coated with microscopic powdered BPA, and which many of us handle daily.

The Panel rejected the March 2009 FDA safety assessment of BPA as "incomplete and unreliable because it failed to consider all the relevant scientific works." The Panel also warned that FDA's "safety assessment on BPA" had been rejected by a March 2009 consortium of independent experts from academia, government, and industry. The Panel report further emphasized that "science at the FDA is deficient, and the Agency is not prepared to meet regulatory responsibilities."

The scientific evidence on the toxic effects of BPA is extensive. A 2007 review of about 700 studies on BPA, published in the journal Reproductive Toxicology, found that the fetus and infants are highly vulnerable to the toxic hormonal effects of this ingredient, technically known as "endocrine disruptive." An accompanying study by National Institutes of Health researchers reported uterine damage in newborn rodents exposed to levels of BPA comparable with those of normal human exposure. This finding may also implicate BPA as a cause of reproductive tract disorders in women, after their earlier exposure as fetuses or infants.

Previous studies in the journal Endocrinology, besides elsewhere, reported that BPA masculinizes the brain of female mice and feminizes the brain of male mice. Toxic effects of this hormone disrupter in pregnant women are evidenced in their infant baby boys by the reduction in the normal distance between their anus and genitals. This decrease in anogenital distance is also associated with a decrease in sperm production. Based on such evidence, Health Canada declared BPA to be a "toxic chemical" in early 2008.

In addition to these toxic effects, exposure of pregnant rodents to BPA, at levels 2,000 times lower than the Environmental Protection Agency's "safe dose," resulted in sexual abnormalities in their offspring. These include an increased number of "terminal end buds" in breast tissue, which are associated with a subsequent high risk of breast cancer. However, an American Plastics Council spokesman claimed that the human relevance of these finding is only "hypothetical."

BPA has also been found in human blood, placental and fetal tissue, and incriminated as a predisposing factor for prostate cancer. The authors of this study also linked endocrine-dependent human cancers, such as breast cancer, to the minimal levels of BPA to which pregnant women are exposed. An August 2, 2007 consensus statement by several dozen scientists warned that BPA, even at very low exposure levels, is probably responsible for many human reproductive disorders.

A September 2008 publication, Endocrine-Related Cancer, by one of us (Dr. Gail Prins) reviewed the substantial scientific evidence on the toxic hormonal effects of BPA, besides other endocrine disruptive chemicals (EDC's) in pregnant women. She concluded that infants and children are highly sensitive to their toxic effects, particularly subsequent risks of prostate cancer.

In October 2008, *Science Daily* reported on an article on BPA called "A Plastic World," in a then pending special section on Environmental Research. Two other articles reported that fetal exposure to BPA disrupted the normal development of the brain and behavior in rats and mice. Other articles have also reported that BPA is massively contaminating the oceans and harming aquatic wildlife.

The June 2009 Endocrine Disruption Act authorized the National Institute of Environmental Health Science "to coordinate" research on hormone disruption to prevent exposure to chemicals "that can undermine the development of children before they are born and cause lifelong impairment of their health and function." This Bill was supported by public health, consumer and children's advocacy groups, and further strengthened by California's Senator Dianne Feinstein's legislation to ban BPA from food and beverage containers. Of major relevance, this legislation has also been endorsed by the April 2010 President's Cancer Panel On "Reducing Environmental Cancer Risk: What We Can Do Now," 2008-2009 Annual Report. This further warns that "to a disturbing extent, babies are born pre-polluted."

There are safe alternatives to BPA. As emphasized in the author's 2009 *Toxic Beauty* book, the recent development of "green chemistry" has encouraged the phase-out of product packaging that relies on petrochemical plastic containers, particularly those containing BPA. These containers are now being replaced with biodegradable substitutes, including recycled paper. Such "green" packaging reduces energy use, greenhouse gases, and non-degradable or poorly degradable wastes currently disposed of in landfills.

In January 2010, the FDA announced an "Update on BPA," with particular reference to its use in food packaging, plastic baby bottles, feeding cups, and metal containers, to avoid childhood exposure. Nevertheless, FDA has still failed to take any regulatory action to this effect. Meanwhile, the industry's Cosmetic Ingredient Review Panel does not even make any reference to BPA in its annual "safety assessments."

In March 2010, Congressmen Bobby Rush and Henry Waxman released a draft of the Toxic Chemicals Safety Act of 2010. The key provisions of this Act include establishment of a program to review and protect children from risks of toxic exposures, including BPA. The passage of this legislation is urgently needed in order to ban BPA from baby bottles, food packaging and other consumer products, especially to prevent any further childhood exposure. One month later, Senator Lautenberg introduced the "Safe Chemicals Act of 2010," aimed at revamping the 34 year-old Toxic Substances Control Act. This is intended to ensure that "those who make the chemicals—ought to be responsible for testing them before they are released to the public." This surely should be the case for BPA.

FRANK CONFLICTS OF INTEREST IN THE NATIONAL CANCER INSTITUTE*

In March 2010, the White House nominated Nobel Laureate Harold Varmus as Director of the National Cancer Institute (NCI).

As a key advisor to President Obama's 2008 Presidential campaign, Varmus was subsequently appointed Co-Chairman of the President's Council of Advisors on Science and Technology. He was previously President of the New York Memorial Sloan-Kettering Cancer Center.

Varmus has a distinguished track record in basic research on cancer treatment. However, as emphasized by the Cancer Prevention Coalition, this is paralleled by lack of familiarity with mounting scientific evidence on cancer prevention. Two decades ago, he claimed, "You can't do experiments to see what causes cancer—it's not an accessible problem, and not the sort of thing scientists can afford to do—everything you do can't be risky."

In 1995, Varmus, then Director of the National Institutes of Health, struck the "reasonable pricing clause," protecting against exorbitant industry profiteering from the sale of drugs, developed with tax payer money. Varmus also gave senior NCI staff free license to consult with the cancer drug industry.

---

* Based on a March 29, 2010 Cancer Prevention Coalition press release endorsed by: Rosalie Bertell, Ph.D., Regent, International Physicians for Humanitarian Medicine, Janette D. Sherman, MD, New York Academy of Sciences, 2009; and Quentin D. Young, MD, Chairman, Health and Medicine Policy Research Group.

In this connection, the 2008 edition of Charity Rating Guide & Watchdog Report listed Dr. Varmus with a compensation package of about $2.7 million. This is the highest compensation of over 500 major non-profit organizations ever monitored.

As a past major recipient of NCI funds for basic genetic research, Varmus warned that "reasonable pricing" clauses, protecting against exorbitant industry profiteering from drugs developed with tax-payer dollars, were driving away private industry. So he struck these from agreements between industry and the NCI. As a consequence, Varmus eliminated any price controls on cancer drugs made at the tax-payer expense.

Illustratively, using taxpayers' money, NCI paid for the research and development of Taxol, an anticancer drug, later manufactured by Bristol-Myers Squibb. Following completion of clinical trials, an extremely expensive process in itself, the public paid again for developing the drug's manufacturing process. Once completed, NCI officials gave Bristol-Myers Squibb the exclusive right to sell Taxol at an inflationary price. As investigative journalist, Joel Bleifuss, warned in a 1995 In These Times article, "Bristol-Myers Squibb sells Taxol to the public for $4.87 per milligram, which is more than 20 times what it costs to produce." Taxol has been a blockbuster for Bristol-Myers, posting sales of over $3 billion since its approval in 1992, and accounting for about 40 percent of the company's sales.

Taxol was not the only drug involved in such funding practices. Bristol-Myers Squibb now sells nearly one-third of the approximately thirty-five cancer drugs currently available, often with highly inflated profits, and often developed with taxpayer funds. In 1995, Varmus, a past major recipient of NCI funds for basic genetic research, decided that "reasonable pricing" clauses, protecting against profiteering from drugs developed with taxpayer dollars, were driving away private industry. So he struck these from pricing clauses.

Taxol was not an isolated example. Taxpayers have funded NCI's research and development for over two-thirds of all cancer drugs now on the market. In a surprisingly frank admission, Samuel Broder, NCI Director from 1989 to 1995, stated the obvious: "The NCI has become what amounts to a government pharmaceutical company." Nobel Laureate Leland Hartwell, President of the Fred Hutchinson Cancer Research Center, endorsed Broder's criticism. He further stressed that most resources for cancer research are spent on "promoting ineffective drugs" for terminal disease. In this connection, Memorial Sloan-Kettering's Leonard Saltz estimated that the price for new biotech drugs "has increased 500-fold in the last decade." Furthermore, the U.S. spends five times more than the U.K. on cancer chemotherapy per patient, although survival rates are similar.

As an expert in cancer treatment, Varmus appears unaware that almost 700 carcinogens, to some of which the public is periodically or regularly exposed, have been identified by independent scientists. He also seems to be unaware that the more cancer is prevented the less there is to treat.

On June 15, 2009, a letter to Congressional leaders urging drastic reform of the Obama Cancer Plan to mandate prevention, besides urging the annual publication of a public registry of carcinogens, was released by the five scientists listed below. This letter also listed seven cancers, summarized their avoidable causes, and their increasing incidence since 1975, based on 2005 NCI data:

- Childhood leukemia has increased by 55% due to ionizing radiation; domestic pesticides; nitrite preservatives in meats, particularly hot dogs; and parental exposures to occupational carcinogens;
- Malignant melanoma (mortality) of the skin in adults has increased by 168% due to the use of sunscreens in childhood that fail to block long wave ultraviolet light;
- Thyroid cancer has increased by 124% due in large part to ionizing radiation;
- Non-Hodgkin's lymphoma has increased by 76% due mostly to phenoxy herbicides; and phenylenediamine hair dyes;
- Testicular cancer has increased by 49% due to pesticides; hormonal ingredients in cosmetics and personal care products; and estrogen residues in meat;
- Ovary cancer (mortality) for women over the age of 65 has increased by 47% in African American women and 13% in Caucasian women due to genital use of talc powder;
- Breast cancer has increased by 17% due to a wide range of factors. These include: birth control pills; toxic hormonal ingredients in cosmetics and personal care products; diagnostic radiation; and routine premenopausal mammography, with a cumulative breast dose exposure of up to about five rads over ten years.

However, and as an expert in cancer treatment, Varmus was unlikely to be aware of such scientific evidence, which was not widely recognized until relatively recently.

Based on recent estimates by the National Institutes of Health, the total costs of cancer are about $219 billion each year. The annual costs to taxpayers of diagnosis and treatment amounts to $89 billion; the annual costs of premature death are conservatively estimated at $112 billion; and the annual costs due to loss of productivity are conservatively estimated at $18 billion.

The human costs surely are of far greater magnitude. Much of these costs could be saved by cancer prevention.

These concerns regarding Dr. Varmus have been recognized and endorsed by the following leading national experts on cancer prevention:

(The Late) Rosalie Bertell, Ph.D.
Regent, International Physicians for Humanitarian Medicine

Janette D. Sherman, MD
New York Academy of Science, 2009

Quentin D. Young, MD
Chairman, Health and Medicine Policy Research Group

CANCER RISKS OF DENTAL AND MEDICAL RADIATION

The longstanding and well-documented evidence on the radiation dangers of premenopausal mammography are persuasive, although belatedly recognized. In striking contrast, evidence on the dangers of routine and highly profitable dental radiation, particularly in children, is still virtually unrecognized, as warned explicitly in my 1978 book, *The Politics of Cancer*.

Dentists are often guilty, and criminally so, of overexposing their patients to radiation dangers. Some dentists require a full set of sixteen to eighteen films every time a patient comes in for a routine checkup. However, the additional diagnostic information furnished by such a series, over and above inspection aided by a dental pick, is difficult to imagine. More conservatively, but still ill-advisably, the American Dental Association recommends that a full set need not be taken more often than every three to five years; and other authorities have extended this to between six and ten years.

These concerns were explicitly emphasized by the late Dr. John Gofman, the leading international authority on the dangers of radiation. In 2001, he published a report warning of the well-documented evidence on the cancer risks to children of alleged "low dose" medical X-rays.

A July 2006 publication by Dr. Ruth Kleinerman in Pediatric Oncology, "Cancer Risks Following Diagnostic and Therapeutic Radiation Exposure in Children," warned that the most radiosensitive organ in children is the thyroid gland. This report also noted that "Although thyroid cancer is rare, 6 other large studies previously confirmed its relationship with prior radiation for treatment of enlarged tonsils or other head, face, or neck concerns."

Furthermore, a report in the U.K. June 2010 *MailOnline* newspaper warned that "Ten dental x-rays raise cancer risks—by at least ten times." This article also cautioned that "X-rays should not be given at routine checkups or when registering new patients, despite these practices still being common in many dental surgeries.

The *MailOnline* report also cited a 2010 collaborative study between the U.K. National Health Service and the universities of Brighton and Sussex. This warned that "multiple exposures to dental X-rays may be associated with increased risks of developing thyroid cancer, particularly in children and adolescents." The report further noted that these findings are consistent with previous warnings of increased risks of thyroid cancer in dentists and their assistants. Further evidence of these risks was published in a November 22, 2010 New York Times article, "Radiation Worries for Children in Dentists' Chairs." This warned against risks of radiation from a new scanning device, known as a cone-beam (CT) scanner. This generates X-ray images, while rotating around the patient, and emits much higher radiation levels than conventional dental X-rays.

Not surprisingly, the incidence of thyroid cancer has escalated by 168% since 1975. The past and continuing practice of routine dental radiation, especially in children, is flagrant malpractice, if not criminal.

A January 3, 2011 *New York Times* article "Study of Children Raised Concerns over Radiation," reported that "the first large study on the use of medical radiation in children says that the average child will get more than seven radiation scans by age 18. Most of them involve X-rays. But there is growing concern about computerized tomography (CT) scans, which entail far more radiation and can raise the risk of cancer. More than 3 percent of children got two or more CT scans. "That's particularly concerning," said Dr. Adam Dorfman of University of Michigan Medical School, the lead author of the study, which appeared Monday in The Archives of Pediatrics and Adolescent Medicine."

A June 7, 2012 National Cancer Institute press release also linked childhood CT scans to leukemia and brain cancer. This study reported that "children and young adults scanned multiple times by CT developed a small risk of leukemia and brain cancer in the decade following first scan." The study also warned that the radiation from a single CT scan "is often up to 10 times higher than that delivered by a conventional x-ray procedure."

A June 12, 2012 *New York Times* article, "Radiation Concerns Rise with Patients' Exposure" reported that the risks of a patient's radiation exposure increased with the rising use of diagnostic imaging like CT scans. This has resulted in a small but significant increase in the risks of leukemia and brain cancer in children. These concerns were confirmed by a June 2012 National Institute of Health study, published in *The Lancet*, based on a study of over 175,000 children and young adults, reported that children and young adults scanned several times by computerized tomography have a "small but significant risk of leukemia and brain cancer" in the following decade. Nevertheless, the study emphasized that the benefits of CT scans should outweigh the risks involved.

CONGRESSIONAL INITIATIVES TO PROTECT CHILDREN AND THE PUBLIC FROM AVOIDABLE CAUSES OF CANCER[*]

The Federal Food, Drug and Cosmetic Act of 1906

Enacted as the nation's first major food and drug law, this was replaced in 1938 by another Act of the same name. This mandates pure and wholesome foods, safe and effective drugs, safe cosmetics, truthful labeling, inspection of drug manufacturing plants every two years, and the testing of drugs, coloring additives and foods chemicals by the FDA.

The Federal Food, Drug and Cosmetic Act of 1938

The Act, enacted in 1906 as the nation's first food and drug law, gave FDA extensive regulatory authority, with particular reference to problems of product safety. This Act was replaced in 1938 by another Act of the same name.

---

[*] Epstein and Grundy. *Consumer Health and Product Hazards/Chemicals Electronic Products, Radiation, Volume 1 of The Legislation of Product Safety*. MIT Press, 1974.

The Public Health Service Act of 1944

This contains 4 sections that were transferred to FDA jurisdiction in 1969. These cover: milk; food and water; sanitary facilities for travelers; sanitary practices in restaurants and food-service establishments; and determining causes and finding means of preventing accidental poisoning and injuries by consumer products.

Federal Insecticide, Fungicide, and Rodenticide Act of 1947

FIFRA regulates the marketing, in interstate commerce, of "economic poisons and devices," which includes insecticides, rodenticides, herbicides, and household disinfectants. It requires registration, appropriate labeling, and in some cases coloring of pesticide products in attempts to protect the user and handler.

The Delaney Amendment to the Food, Drug and Cosmetic Act of 1958

This prohibits the use of any carcinogenic chemical as a food additive. Specifically, the law states: "That no additive shall be deemed safe if it is found to induce cancer when ingested by man or animal, or if it is found, after tests which are appropriate for the evaluation of the safety of food additives, to induce cancer in man or animal . . ."

The Federal Hazardous Substances Act of 1960

Originally known as the Federal Hazardous Substances Labeling Act, this Act is administered by the Bureau of Product Safety of the FDA. The Act covers all categories of household products, including toys, but not the raw materials from which they are manufactured.

The Act was based on the recognition of the potential hazards of some consumer products, and on the belief that certain hazards may be minimized or prevented by cautionary labeling. Their hazards and also the penalties for violation or omission must be stated on the label. The labels must also include the words "Danger" for highly toxic substances, and "Warning" or "Caution" for all other ingredients.

The Child Protection Act of 1966

This Act bans from interstate commerce toys and articles so hazardous that adequate warnings could not be written. The Act strengthens the

Hazardous Substances Act of 1960 and prevents the marketing of potentially harmful toys. The Child Protection and Toy Safety Act of 1969 amends the Federal Hazardous Substances Act to protect children from articles which contain thermal, electrical or mechanical hazards.

The Fair Packaging and Labeling Act of 1966

This requires complete and prominent labeling information on packages and containers to aid shoppers in comparing values and to prevent deceptive packaging practices. FDA jurisdiction extends to the packaging of foods, drugs, medical devices and cosmetics.

The Radiation Control for Healthy and Safety Act of 1968

This protects the public from unnecessary exposure to radiation from electronic products.

Child Protection and Toy Safety Act of 1969

This amends the Federal Hazardous Substances Act to protect children from toys and other articles which contain thermal, electrical or mechanical hazards.

The Poison Prevention Packaging Act of 1970

This requires special packaging of potentially dangerous household goods to protect children from serious illness (including cancer) resulting from accidental handling, using, or eating such substances. This is designed to protect children from accidentally eating toxic substances by requiring special packaging which children under five have trouble opening, while adults would not.

The Consumer Product Safety Act of 1972

Signed into law in 1972, it established a Consumer Product Safety Commission (CPSC), which represented a dramatic step forward in efforts to protect the consumer against "unreasonable injuries" associated with consumer products. Authorities transferred to the CPSC were principally those administered by the FDA's Bureau of Product Safety. These statutes included:

1. The Federal Hazardous Substances Labeling Act of 1960
2. The Child Protection Act of 1966
3. The Poison Prevention Packaging Act of 1970.

The Poison Prevention Packaging Act, enacted in 1970, was designed to protect children from accidentally eating toxic substances by requiring special packaging designed so that children under five would have trouble opening a package, while adults would not.

Toxic Substances Control Act (TSCA) of 1976

The Act provides the Environmental Protection Agency (EPA) with authority to require reporting, record-keeping, record-keeping and testing requirements, and restrictions relating to chemical substances and/or mixtures. Certain substances are generally excluded from TSCA, including, among others, food, drugs, cosmetics and pesticides. TSCA addresses the production, importation, use, and disposal of specific chemicals including polychlorinated biphenyls, asbestos, radon and lead-based paint.

The Safe Chemicals Act of 2012

This Act modernizes the 1976 Toxic Substances Control Act (TSCA). It requires chemical companies to demonstrate the safety of their industrial chemicals, and the EPA to evaluate the chemicals' safety based on the best available science.

CANCER PREVENTION COALITION CITIZEN PETITIONS TO THE FDA, 1995-2007

November 17, 1994	Seeking Carcinogenic Labeling On All Cosmetic Talc Products
January 17, 1995	Seeking To Ban The Use Of Lindane As Treatment For Lice And Scabies
April 25, 1995	Seeking Labeling Of Nitrite-Preserved Hot Dogs For Childhood Cancer Risk
October 22, 1996	Seeking Cancer Warning On Cosmetics and Personal Care Products Containing DEA
May 11, 2007	Seeking the Withdrawal of the New Animal Drug Application Approval for Genetically-Engineered (rBGH) Milk
January 29, 2010	Imminent Health Hazard from Hormonal Meat

SEEKING CARCINOGENIC LABELING ON ALL COSMETIC TALC PRODUCTS

November 17, 1994

David A. Kessler, M.D.
Commissioner
Food and Drug Administration, Room 1-23
12420 Parklawn Drive
Rockville, MD 20857

The undersigned submits on behalf of the Cancer Prevention Coalition, Inc. (CPC), Samuel S. Epstein, M.D., Chair and National Advisor of the Ovarian Cancer Early Detection and Prevention Foundation (OCEDPF), Nancy Nehls Nelson, member of the Ovarian Cancer Early Detection and Prevention Foundation, Peter Orris, M.D. and Quentin Young, M.D. This citizen petition is based on scientific papers dating back to the 1960s which warn of increased cancer rates resulting from frequent exposure to cosmetic grade talc.

The undersigned submits this petition under 21 U.S.C. 321 (n), 361, 362, and 371 (a); and 21 CFR 740.1, 740.2 of 21 CFR 10.30 of the Federal Food, Drug, and Cosmetic Act to request the Commissioner of Food and Drugs to require that all cosmetic talc products bear labels with a warning such as Talcum powder causes cancer in laboratory animals. Frequent talc application in the female genital area increases risk of ovarian cancer.

A. AGENCY ACTION REQUESTED

This petition requests that FDA take the following action:

1. Immediately require cosmetic talcum powder products to bear labels with a warning such as Talcum powder causes cancer in laboratory animals. Frequent talc application in the female genital area increases the risk of ovarian cancer.
2. Pursuant to 21 CFR 10.30 (h) (2), a hearing at which time we can present our scientific evidence.

B. STATEMENT OF GROUNDS

Ovarian cancer is the fourth deadliest women's cancer in the U.S., striking approximately 23,000 and killing approximately 14,000 women this year.

Ovarian cancer is very difficult to detect at the early stages of the disease, making the survival rate very low. Only three percent of ovarian cancer cases can be attributed to family history. One of the avoidable risk factors for ovarian cancer is the daily use of talcum powder in the genital area.

Research done as early as 1961 has shown that particles, similar to talc and asbestos particles, can translocate from the exterior genital area to the ovaries in women. These findings provide support to the unexpected high rate of mortality from ovarian cancer in female asbestos workers. Minute particles, such as talc are able to translocate through the female reproductive tract and cause foreign body reactions in the ovary.

There is a large body of scientific evidence, dating back thirty years, on the toxicity and mineralogy of cosmetic talc products. As early as 1968, Cralley et al. Concluded:

> All of the 22 talcum products analyzed have a . . . fiber content . . . averaging 19%. The fibrous material was predominantly talc but probably contained minor amounts of tremolite, anthophyllite, and chrysotile [asbestos-like fibers] as these are often present in fibrous talc mineral deposits . . . Unknown significant amounts of such materials in products that may be used without precautions may create an unsuspected problem.

As a follow-up to previous findings, Rohl, et al., examined 21 samples of consumer talcums and powders, including baby powders, body powders, facial powders and pharmaceutical powders between 1971-1975. The study concluded:

> ". . . cosmetic grade talc was not used exclusively. The presence in these products of asbestiform anthophyllite and tremolite, chrysotile, and quartz indicates the need for a regulatory standard for cosmetic talc . . . We also recommend that evaluation be made to determine the possible health hazards associated with the use of these products."

Talc is a carcinogen, with or without the presence of asbestos-like fibers. In 1993, the National Toxicology Program published a study on the toxicity of non-asbestiform talc and found clear evidence of carcinogenic activity.

Recent cancer research in the United States has found conclusively that frequent talcum powder application in the genital area increases a woman's risk of developing ovarian cancer. Cramer, et al, suggested that talc application directly to the genital area around the time of ovulation might lead to talc particles becoming deeply imbedded in the substance of the ovary and perhaps causing foreign body reaction (granulomas) capable of causing growth of epithelial ovarian tissue.

Harlow, et al, found that frequent talc use directly on the genital area during ovulation increased a woman's risk **threefold.** That study also found:

> "The most frequent method of talc exposure was use as a dusting powder directly to the perineum (genitals) . . . Brand or generic 'baby powder' was used most frequently and was the category associated with a statistically significant risk for ovarian cancer."

In Harlow's report, arguably the most comprehensive study of talc use and ovarian cancer to date, 235 ovarian cancer cases were identified and compared to 239 controls, women with no sign of ovarian cancer or related health problems. Through personal interviews, Harlow, et al, found that 16.7% of the control group reported frequent talc application to the perineum. This percentage is useful in estimating the number of women in the general population exposed to cosmetic talc in the genital area on a regular basis. Harlow, et al, concludes:

> ". . . given the poor prognosis for ovarian cancer, any potentially harmful exposures should be avoided, particularly those with limited benefits. For this reason, we discourage the use of talc in genital hygiene, particularly as a daily habit."

Clearly, large numbers of women—an estimated 17%—are using cosmetic talc in the genital area and may not be adequately warned of the risk of ovarian cancer from daily use.

C. CLAIM FOR CATEGORICAL EXCLUSION

A claim for categorical exclusion is asserted pursuant to 21 CFR 25.24 (a) (11).

D. CERTIFICATION

The undersigned certifies, that, to the best knowledge and belief of the undersigned, this petition includes all information and views on which the petition relies, and that it includes representative data and information known to the petitioner which are unfavorable to the petition.

This petition is submitted by:

Jill A. Cashen

Samuel S. Epstein, M.D.
Cancer Prevention Coalition

Michael E. Deutsch, Legal Director
Center for Constitutional Rights

APPENDIX I: Results for an informal survey of talc products in Chicago drug stores.

BABY POWDERS

Johnson & Johnson Baby Powder. Contains: TALC, fragrance.

Osco Brand Baby Powder. Contains: TALC, fragrance.

Jean Nate Perfumed Talc. Contains: TALC, kaolin, magnesium carbonate, fragrance.

Shower to Shower. Contains: TALC, cornstarch, sodium bicarbonate, fragrance, polysaccharides.

Ammens Medicated Powder. Contains: Zinc oxide, cornstarch, fragrance, isostearic acid, PPG-20, methyl glucose ether, TALC.

Cashmere Bouquet Perfumed Powder. Contains: TALC, magnesium carbonate, zinc stearate, fragrance.

Gold Bond Medicated Powder. Contains: Menthol, zinc oxide, boric acid, eucalyptol, methyl salicylate, salicylic acid, TALC, thymol, zinc stearate.

FEMININE PRODUCTS

Vagisil Feminine Powder. Contains: Cornstarch, aloe, mineral oil, magnesium stearate, silica, benzethonium chloride, fragrance.

Vaginex Feminine Powder. Contains: Zinc oxide, cornstarch, fragrance, 6-hydroxquinoline, 8-hydroxquinoline sulfate, isostearic acid, PPG-20, methyl glucose ether, TALC.

Summer's Eve Feminine Powder. Contains: Cornstarch, tricalcium phosphate, oxoxynol-9, benzethonium chloride, fragrance.

FDS Feminine Deodorant Spray. Contains: Isobutane, isopropyl myristate, cornstarch, mineral oil, fragrance, lanolin alcohol, hydrated silica, magnesium stearate, benzyl alcohol.

SEEKING TO BAN THE USE OF LINDANE FOR TREATING LICE AND SCABIES

January 17, 1995

David A. Kessler, M.D.
Commissioner
Food and Drug Administration, Room 1-23
12420 Parklawn Drive
Rockville, MD 2085 7

The undersigned submits on behalf of the Cancer Prevention Coalition, Inc. (CPC), Samuel S. Epstein, M.D., Chair, Quentin Young, M.D., and Peter Orris, M.D., and on behalf of the Center for Constitutional Rights, Michael Deutsch, Esq. This citizen petition is based on recent scientific information on risks of brain cancer in children resulting from the use of lindane shampoo, other evidence of carcinogenicity, and evidence of haematotoxicity and neurotoxicity.

The undersigned submits this petition under 21 U.S.C. 321 (n), 361, 362, and 371 (a); and 21 CFR 740.1, 740.2 of 21 CFR 10.30 of the Federal Food, Drug, and Cosmetic Act to request the Commissioner of the Food and Drug Administration (FDA) to immediately ban the use of lindane as a treatment for lice and scabies.

A. AGENCY ACTION REQUESTED

This petition requests that FDA take the following action:
Immediately ban the use of lindane as a treatment for lice and scabies.
Pursuant to 21 CFR 10.30 (h) (2), a hearing at which time we can present our scientific evidence.

B. STATEMENT OF GROUNDS

Lice and scabies are endemic among the population. An estimated six million Americans, mainly children, are infested with lice each year. Most children are treated with pesticide-containing products marketed as shampoos. Lindane (gamma-hexachlorocyclohexane) is one of the most widely prescribed treatments for lice and scabies.

In a recent case-control study, Davis, et al. reported a statistically significant increase of brain cancer in children following treatment with lindane shampoo.

> ". . . use of Kwell®, [lindane] was significantly associated with childhood brain cancer in comparison to friend controls (OR = 4.6; 95% CI = 1.0-21.3)."

These findings are of particular significance in relation to the striking increase, 38%, in the incidence of brain and nervous system cancers in children from 1973-1991.

Further evidence on carcinogenicity is provided by two epidemiological studies by the National Cancer Institute. Statistically significant increases, up to six-fold, in the incidence of non-Hodgkin's lymphoma were reported in farmers exposed to lindane.

In addition to these epidemiological data, series of case reports on blood disorders, including aplastic anemia, with case fatality rates of some 50%, and leukemia have appeared in the literature over the last three decades. Of related interest is recent evidence on the high toxicity of lindane to human red blood stem cells.

These epidemiological data are further supported by experimental evidence on the carcinogenicity of lindane. Lindane is classified as Group 2B by the International Agency for Research on Cancer, and as 2B/C by the Environmental Protection Agency. The EPA has restricted lindane's use as an agricultural pesticide. Agricultural and other uses of lindane and other isomers of hexachlorocyclohexane have been severely restricted or banned by other countries.

The neurotoxic effects of lindane are well known. A 1976 FDA alert was issued to warn physicians of such risks. Numerous case reports have documented seizures and brain damage following lindane exposure. Recent studies have emphasized that recommended dosages of lindane may cause seizures:

> "Therefore, given the extremely narrow range of safety of this drug and the risk imposed by the kindling effects, which potentiates convulsive seizures, and that this potentiation may be carried on for a considerable period of time, there is no good reason to use lindane in children or adults when other perfectly effective, safer pediculides are available."

Lindane is readily absorbed through the skin. After topical application to the adult skin without washing for 24 hours, almost 10% can be recovered from urine. Absorption is further increased when lindane is administered in warm water or followed by oil-based hair care preparations.

C. CLAIM FOR CATEGORICAL EXCLUSION

A Claim for categorical exclusion is asserted pursuant to 21 CFR 25.24 (a) (11).

D. CERTIFICATION

The undersigned certifies, that, to the best knowledge and belief of the undersigned, this petition includes all information and views on which the petition relies, and that it includes representative data and information known to the petitioner which are unfavorable to the petition.

This petition, supported by 15 scientific references, remains ignored by the FDA.

Samuel S. Epstein, M.D.
Chairman, Cancer Prevention Coalition
Professor emeritus Occupational and Environmental Medicine
University of Illinois School of Public Health, Chicago

Quentin D. Young, M.D.
Chairman, Health and Medicine Policy Research Group
Past President of the American Public Health Association

Peter Orris, M.D.
Professor and Chief of Service
University of Illinois at Chicago Medical Center

Michael Deutsch, Esq.
Legal Director, Center for Constitutional Rights, New York

SEEKING LABELING OF NITRITE-PRESERVED HOT DOGS FOR CHILDHOOD CANCER RISK

April 25, 1995

David A. Kessler, M.D.
Commissioner, Food and Drug Administration, Room 1-23
12420 Parklawn Drive
Rockville, MD 20857

The undersigned submits on behalf of the Cancer Prevention Coalition, Inc. (CPC), Samuel S. Epstein, M.D., Chair, and on behalf of the Center for constitutional Rights, Michael Deutsch, Esq., Legal Director. This citizen petition is based on accumulating scientific information on excess risks of childhood brain tumors and leukemia from the consumption of hot dogs containing nitrite preservatives.

The undersigned submits this petition under 21 U.S.C. 321 (n), 361, 362, and 371 (a); and 21 CFR 740.1, 740.2 of 21 CFR 10.30 of the Federal Food, Drug, and Cosmetic Act to request the Commissioner of the Food and Drug Administration (FDA) to label hot dogs that contain nitrites with a cancer risk warning.

A. AGENCY ACTION REQUESTED

This petition requests that FDA take the following action:
Immediately require nitrite-containing hot dogs to be labeled with warnings such as hot dogs containing nitrites have been shown to pose risks of childhood cancer. Pursuant to 21 CFR 10.30 (h) (2), a hearing at which time we can present our scientific evidence.

B. STATEMENT OF GROUNDS

Nitrites are widely used as preservatives in hot dogs, besides other meat products. Nitrites combine with amines naturally present in meat to form carcinogenic N-nitroso compounds. N-nitrosodimethylamine has been identified in nitrite-preserved meat products. (There is overwhelming evidence on the carcinogenicity of N-nitrosodimmethylamine in animal experiments. Furthermore, epidemiologic evidence has associated N-nitroso carcinogens with cancer of the oral cavity, urinary bladder, esophagus, stomach and brain.

There is substantial evidence on the risks of childhood cancer from the consumption of meats containing nitrites. In 1982, Preston-Martin, et al. found that consumption during pregnancy of meats cured with sodium nitrite has been associated with development of brain tumors in the offspring.

Recent case-control studies have confirmed the risks of cancer from consumption of hot dogs. Eating many hot dogs by children, as well maternal hot dog consumption during pregnancy, has been shown to be associated with brain cancer and leukemia in children.

Bunin, et al. studied children who were diagnosed with brain cancer before age six, between 1986 and 1989. Of 53 foods and beverages and three alcoholic beverages consumed by mothers during pregnancy, only hot dogs were associated with an excess risk of childhood brain tumor.

Sarusua and Savitz studied 234 childhood cancer cases in Denver and found a strong association between the consumption of hot dogs and brain cancer. Children born to mothers who consumed hot dogs one or more times per week during pregnancy had approximately double the risk of developing brain tumors. Children who ate hot dogs one or more times per week were also at higher risk of brain cancer. In addition, children who ate hot dogs and took no vitamins, which retard the formation of N-nitroso carcinogens, were more strongly associated with both acute lymphocytic leukemia (ALL) and brain cancer.

Peters and his colleagues studied the relationship between eating certain foods and the risk of leukemia in children from birth to age 10 in Los Angeles County between 1980 and 1987. The researchers found that children who ate 12 or more hot dogs per month were found to have approximately nine times the normal risk for developing childhood leukemia. A strong risk for childhood leukemia also existed for those children whose fathers' intake of hot dogs was 12 or more per month. Peters, et al. concluded:

"Our results provide evidence for an association between consumption of hot dogs and risk of childhood leukemia. Adjustments for all factors thought to be potential confounders did not affect these associations. Independent risks were associated with both children's and fathers' consumption . . . The findings, if correct, suggest that reduced consumption of hot dogs could reduce leukemia risks, especially in those consuming the most."

These findings are of particular significance considering a 38 percent increase in the incidence of brain and nervous system cancers in children from 1973-1991. Brain tumors account for about one in five childhood cancers.

C. CLAIM FOR CATEGORICAL EXCLUSION

A claim for categorical exclusion is asserted pursuant to 21 CFR 25.24 (a) (11).

D. CERTIFICATION

The undersigned certifies, that, to the best knowledge and belief of the undersigned, this petition includes all information and views on which the petition relies, and that it includes representative data and information known to the petitioner which are unfavorable to the petition.

This petition, supported by 24 scientific references, remains ignored by the FDA.

Samuel S. Epstein, M.D.
Chairman, Cancer Prevention Coalition
Professor Occupational and Environmental Medicine
University of Illinois at Chicago

Michael Deutsch, Esq.
Legal Director, Center for Constitutional Rights, New York

SEEKING CANCER WARNING ON COSMETICS AND PERSONAL CARE PRODUCTS CONTAINING DEA

October 22, 1996

David A. Kessler, M.D.
Commissioner
Food and Drug Administration
Room #14-71
Rockville, MD 20857

The undersigned submits on behalf of the Cancer Prevention Coalition, Inc., and its Chairman, Samuel S. Epstein, M.D., and on behalf of the Center for Constitutional Rights, Michael Deutsch, Esquire. This petition is based on scientific evidence of increased cancer risks from exposure to nitrosamines in cosmetics.

The undersigned submits this petition, under 21 U.S.C. 321 (n), 361, 362 and 371 (a); and 21 CFR 740.1, 740.2 of 21 CFR 10.30 of the Federal Food, Drug, and Cosmetic Act, to the Commissioner of Food and Drugs requiring that all cosmetic products containing diethanolamine (DEA) bear labels with a warning: "Caution—This product may contain N-nitrosodiethanolamine, a known cancer-causing agent."

A. AGENCY ACTION REQUESTED

This petition requests that FDA takes the following action:

(1) Issue a regulation under the Federal Food, Drug and Cosmetic Act, Section 601(a), stating that "All cosmetics containing diethanolamine (DEA), a constituent of diethanolamide soaps that may react with nitrosating agents to form N-nitrosodiethanolamine (NDEA), bear a label as an adulterated product containing poisonous and deleterious substances which may render it injurious to users under the conditions of use prescribed in the labeling thereof, or under such conditions of use as are customary or usual: that which contains DEA also bears the following legend conspicuously displayed thereon: 'Caution—This product may contain N-nitrosodi-ethanolamine (NDEA), a known cancer-causing agent.'"

(2) For purposes of enforcement of this act, the Secretary should conduct examinations and investigations of products which may be contaminated with NDEA through regular and routine analytical

testing by officers and employees of the Department or through any health, food, or drug officer or employee of any State, Territory or political subdivision thereof, duly commissioned by the Secretary of the Department. Such examinations should result in removal of products from the shelves if products do not comply with labeling regulations.
(3) Pursuant to 21 CFR 10.30 (h) (2), a hearing at which time we can present our scientific evidence.

B. STATEMENT OF GROUNDS

1. *Widespread Contamination of Cosmetics with DEA and NDEA*

Diethanolamine (DEA) is a high production chemical used in a wide range of cosmetic pro-ducts, including shampoos, lotions and creams. In the presence of long-chain fatty acids DEA reacts to form neutral ethanolamide soaps, which are used as wetting agents in cosmetics. These soaps contain unreacted DEA. Triethanolamine (TEA), also used widely in cosmetics, may also be contaminated with DEA. According to the Cosmetics, Toiletries and Fragrance Association,

Cocamide DEA, Lauramide DEA, Linoleamide DEA and Oleamide DEA are fatty acid diethanolamides which may contain 4 to 33 percent diethanolamine. These ingredients are used in cosmetics at concentrations of <0.1 percent to 50 percent, with most products containing 1 percent to 25 percent diethanolamide.

As of 1980, FDA reported that approximately 42 percent of all cosmetic products were contaminated with NDEA at the following concentrations: facial cosmetics from .042 to 49 mg/kg, lotions from less than .010 to .140 mg/kg, shampoos from less than 10 to 160 mg/kg. In two surveys of cosmetics, 27 out of 29 American products contained up to 48 mg/kg NDEA. A more recent FDA analysis (1991-1992) found that NDEA is present in some products at mg/kg concentrations.

2. *DEA Is a Precursor of NDEA*

N-nitrosodiethanolamine (NDEA), is readily formed in cosmetic by nitrosation of DEA. Even small amounts of DEA in cosmetics can react with nitrosating agents to form nitrosamines. According to the Cosmetics, Toiletries and Fragrance Association: Nitrosamine contamination of diethanolamine and fatty acid diethanolamides, and nitrosamine formation are potential problems in using these diethanolamides. The diethanolamides used in cosmetic products should be free of nitrosamines, and the finished product should not contain nitrosating agents as ingredients.

Nitrosating agents are added to cosmetics in one of three ways: (a) Nitrites are added directly as anti-corrosive agents; (b) Nitrites are released by the degradation of 2-nitro-1,3-propanediol (BNDP); and (c) Nitrites are contaminants in the raw materials or resulting from the exposure of cosmetics to air. Secondary amines, such as DEA, are rapidly nitrosated by nitrogen oxides. Nitrosamines formation from nitrite and amines is accelerated under specific conditions by formaldehyde, paraformaldehyde, thiocyanate, nitrophenols and certain metal salts (e.g ZnI_2, $CuCl$, $AgNO_3$, $SnCl_2$ and $HgCl_2$).

Cosmetics remain on store shelves and in cabinets of consumers for long periods of time, allowing nitrosamines to form. If DEA is present, nitrosamines can continue to form throughout storage, especially at elevated temperatures.

Acidic pH is an optimal reaction condition for nitrosamine formation. Although cosmetics generally have neutral pH, N-nitrosamines can be formed at neutral or alkaline pH by the reaction of a nitrosating agent with an amine in the presence of carbonyl compounds such as formaldehyde. Formaldehyde is present in cosmetics either from in situ formaldehyde-releasing agents, such as BNDP, or from its use as a preservative.

3. *Dermal Absorption of NDEA*

There is substantial evidence of the dermal absorption of NDEA in both rodents and humans. "[NDEA] is a known carcinogen in laboratory animals; it is absorbed through the skin. The absorption rate is a function of the nature of the cosmetic; absorption is fastest in nonpolar vehicles ". Dermal absorption of NDEA was demonstrated by Lijinsky et al. In 1981. As a fat-soluble chemical NDEA can be absorbed dermally in rats and humans.

4. *NDEA Increases Cancer Risk*

There is substantial evidence of potent carcinogenicity of NDEA in a wide range of animal species. According to the International Agency for Research on Cancer (IARC).

There is sufficient evidence of a carcinogenic effect of N-nitrosodiethanolamine—In view of the widespread exposure to appreciable concentrations of N-nitrosodiethanol-amine, efforts should be made to obtain epidemiological information.

The National Toxicology Program similarly concluded: There is sufficient evidence for the carcinogenicity of N-nitrosodiethanolamine in experimental animals. Of over 44 different species in which N-nitroso compounds have been tested, all have been susceptible. Humans are most unlikely to be the only exception to this trend.

In 1978, the IARC concluded that "although no epidemiological data were available, nitrosodiethanolamine should be regarded for practical purposes as if it were carcinogenic to humans". In 1987 the IARC further confirmed the carcinogenicity of NDEA.

Based on early evidence of the carcinogenicity of NDEA and evidence of cutting fluid contamination, 20 years ago NIOSH recommended that action be taken to protect workers including elimination of nitrosamines from the fluids. More recently, NIOSH published a hazard review of cutting fluids used in metal working that contain NDEA among other nitrosamines. This hazard review indicates that, based on epidemiological evidence in human beings, "Increased cancer risk has been generally attributed to worker exposure to nitrosamine or PAH (polyaromatic hydrocarbon) contaminants in metal working fluids".

5. *The Failure of the FDA to Take Appropriate Regulatory Action*

In the Federal Register of April 10, 1979, the FDA called for industry "to take immediate measures to eliminate to the extent possible [NDEA] and any other N-nitrosamines from cosmetic products," and further insisted that "cosmetic products may be analyzed by FDA for nitrosamine contamination and that individual products could be subject to enforcement action."

FDA has taken no subsequent enforcement actions despite the limited compliance with this Federal Register order. According to the FDA officials Don Havery and Hardy Chou in 1994.

In the United States . . . the personal care industry has invested resources in understanding both the mechanisms of N-nitrosamine formation in cosmetic systems and the means of inhibiting N-nitrosamine formation. However, there is still room for improvement. New products containing nitrosatable amines with formaldehyde and nitrite-releasing preservatives are still appearing on the U.S. market. Manufacturers have a responsibility to be aware of the potential for N-nitrosamine formation and to take steps necessary to keep N-nitrosamine levels as low as possible as part of their good manufacturing practices.

The goal of good manufacturing practices is to reduce "human exposure to N-nitrosamines to the lowest level technologically feasible by reducing levels in all personal care products. With the information and technology currently available to cosmetic manufacturers, N-nitrosamine levels can and should be further reduced in consumer products ".

The FDA has failed to act on the Federal Register recommendations made in 1979. More recently, the FDA has not fully recognized the consumer hazards of this carcinogen. Measurements have not been made to determine total daily exposure to nitrosamines and it is inappropriate to quantify exposures without such data.

6. *Cosmetic Industry Response to FDA Action*

In response to the FDA Federal Register order, the Nitrosamine Task Force of the Cosmetics, Toiletries and Fragrance Association failed to eliminate the use of DEA, but rather, they investigated ways to inhibit the formation of NDEA.

There are no known nitrosation inhibitors that eliminate nitrosamine contamination. Inhibitors have failed for the following reasons:

The compound a-tocopherol has been used as an inhibitor but this compound is useful only when the nitrosating agent is nitrite itself. It is not effective against nitrogen oxide, a gas found in polluted air. It has also been shown to be ineffective in some cosmetic systems.

Many cosmetics make inhibition of nitrosamine formation more difficult. If they are two-phase emulsion systems the inhibitor must be soluble in both hydrophilic and hydrophobic media to be effective as an inhibitor.

Ascorbic acid, sodium bisulfite, butylated hydroxyanisole (BHA), butylated hydroxytoluene (BHT) sodium ascorbated, ascorbyl palmitate and a-tocopherol have all been used in attempts to inhibit nitrosamine formation. None of these inhibitors have been adequate against all possible nitrosation agents to which a shelved cosmetic is exposed.

Industry has had no success in reducing NDEA below 1984 levels. As a result, in 1996 the Cosmetics, Toiletries and Fragrance Association stated in 1996, "These chemicals [Cocamide DEA, Lauramide DEA, Linoleamide DEA, and Oleamide DEA] should not be used as ingredients in cosmetic products containing nitrosating agents". Nevertheless, DEA is still widely used by major cosmetic manufacturers.

In contrast, some other manufacturers such as Aubrey Organics 7, have ceased to use diethanolamide soaps entirely. According to Aubrey Hampton of Aubrey Organics7, None of our products perform less effectively because they do not contain DEA. There are many alternative soap bases available without DEA that can be used by cosmetic manufacturers. In short, the removal of DEA does not pose a manufacturing problem to the cosmetic industry. There is no reason for high levels of NDEA to be found in cosmetic products. With safe alternatives available, the elimination of DEA should not be an economic burden for the cosmetic industry.

7. *Response of National Institutes for Occupational Safety and Health*

In striking contrast to the FDA's position on NDEA, The National Institutes for Occupational Safety and Health (NIOSH) has issued two reports, one as early as 1976, stating that protective measures should be taken when workers are exposed to levels of NDEA similar to those found in cosmetics.

8. *Response of German Industry and European Union*

The German Federal Health Office issued a request to eliminate all secondary amines from cosmetics in 1987 and in response, the German manufacturers 'association has voluntarily complied and sharply reduced the use of secondary amines in cosmetics and toiletries. Included in the specifications of the German Federal Health Office were that fatty acid diethanolamides contain as low as achievable contamination by unreacted diethanolamine. Eisenbrand et al. explained:
Commercially available products from the German market analyzed six to 18 months after the recommendation had been issued showed that only 15 percent were contaminated with [NDEA] or NDHPA . . . . The overall results of this study demonstrate however, a strong downward trend in both levels and frequency of contamination. They prove that nitrosamine contamination of cosmetics can be minimized by simple preventive measures.
The European Union has stated specific maximum allowable concentrations of inadvertently formed N-nitrosodialkanolamine. In legislation that was most recently amended in 1993, the European Union asserted that monoalkanolamines and trialkanolamines must be stored in nitrite free containers, cannot be used in nitrosating systems, must have purity of at least 99% and can contain no more than .5% secondary alkanolamine. With regards to N-nitrosodialkanolamine specifically, the maximum content that the EU allows is 50 micrograms per kilogram (50ppb). In comparison, U.S. cosmetic levels for NDEA as high as 2,960 parts per billion were reported in 1992.

9. *Conclusion*

There is strong evidence proving: the widespread use of DEA in cosmetics, nitrosation of DEA to form NDEA, contamination of cosmetics with NDEA, the potent carcinogenicity of NDEA, and the availability of alternatives to DEA. The FDA should take prompt action to require labels on all products containing DEA that reads: "Caution—This product may contain N-nitrosodi-ethanolamine, a known cancer-causing agent."

C. CLAIM FOR CATEGORICAL EXCLUSION

A claim for categorical exclusion is asserted pursuant to 21 CFR 25.24 (a)(11).

D. CERTIFICATION

The undersigned certifies, that, to the best knowledge and belief of the undersigned, this petition includes all information and views on which the petition relies, and that it includes representative data and information known to the petitioner which are unfavorable to the petition.

This petition, supported by 51 scientific references, was ignored by the FDA.

Samuel S. Epstein, M.D.
Chairman, Cancer Prevention Coalition
Professor Occupational and Environmental Medicine
University of Illinois School of Public Health, Chicago

Michael Deutsch, Esq.
Legal Director, Center for Constitutional Rights, New York

SEEKING THE WITHDRAWAL OF THE NEW ANIMAL DRUG APPLICATION APPROVAL FOR GENETICALLY-ENGINEERED (rBGH) MILK

May 11, 2007

Mike Leavitt
Secretary of Health and Human Services
U.S. Department of Health and Human Services

Andrew C. von Eschenbach, M.D.
Commissioner of Food and Drugs

Dockets Management Branch
Food and Drug Administration, Room 1061
5630 Fishers Lane
Rockville, MD 20852

 The undersigned submits this petition on behalf of the Cancer Prevention Coalition, Samuel S. Epstein, M.D., Chair; the Organic Consumers Association, Ronnie Cummins, Executive Director; Family Farm Defenders, John Kinsman, President; Arpad Pusztai, PhD, FRSE; and Institute for Responsible Technology, Jeffrey M. Smith, Executive Director.
 This petition is based on scientific evidence of increased risks of cancer, particularly breast, colon, and prostate, from the consumption of milk from cows injected with Posilac®, the genetically modified recombinant bovine growth hormone (also known as rBGH, sometribove, recombinant bovine somatotropin, or rbST). Posilac® is the trademark for Monsanto's rBGH product, registered with the U.S. Patent and Trademark Office, and is approved for marketing by the Food and Drug Administration (FDA). This petition is also based on abnormalities in the composition of rBGH milk, resulting from the recognized veterinary toxicity of rBGH, particularly increased levels of IGF-1.
 The undersigned submit this petition under section 512(e)(1) of the Federal Food, Drug, and Cosmetic Act (21 U.S.C. 360b(e)(1)(A)), to request the Secretary to immediately suspend approval of Posilac® based on imminent hazard; and under section 21 U.S.C. 321 (n), 361, 362, and 371 (a), 21 CFR 740.1, 740.2 of 21 CFR 10.30 of the Federal Food, Drug, and Cosmetic Act to request the Commissioner of the Food and Drug Administration to label milk and other dairy products produced with the use of Posilac® with a cancer risk warning.

A. AGENCY ACTION REQUESTED

This petition requests the Secretary and the Commissioner to take the following action:

Suspend approval of Posilac®, and/or require milk and other dairy products produced with the use of Posilac® to be labeled with warnings such as, "Produced with the use of Posilac®, and contains elevated levels of IGF-1, a major risk factor for breast, prostate, and colon cancers."

B. STATEMENT OF GROUNDS

1. *The Veterinary Toxicity of Posilac®*

Evidence of these toxic effects was first detailed in confidential Monsanto reports, based on records of secret nationwide rBGH veterinary trials, submitted to the FDA prior to October 1989 when they were leaked to one of the petitioners, Dr. Epstein then made these reports available to Congressman John Conyers, Chairman of the House Committee on Government Operations. On May 8, 1990, Congressman Conyers issued the following statement. "I find it reprehensible that Monsanto and the FDA have chosen to suppress and manipulate animal health test data." Details of these toxic effects were subsequently admitted by Monsanto and the FDA, and disclosed on the drug's veterinary label (Posilac®) in November, 1993. These include injection site lesions, a wide range of other toxic effects, and an increased incidence of mastitis, requiring the use of medication and antibiotics, and resulting in their contamination of milk.

2. *Abnormalities in rBGH Milk*

In a Monsanto Executive Summary, "Posilac, January 1994," it was claimed that "natural milk is indistinguishable" from rBGH milk and that "There is no legal basis requiring its labeling." However, there are a wide range of well-documented abnormalities in rBGH milk, apart from increased IGF-1 levels. These include: reduction in casein; reduction in short-chain fatty acid and increase in long-chain fatty acid levels; increase in levels of the thyroid hormone triiodothyronine enzyme; contamination with unapproved drugs from treating mastitis; and frequency of pus cells due to mastitis.

3. *Increased Levels of IGF-1 in rBGH Milk*

A wide range of publications have documented excess levels of IGF-1 in rBGH milk, with increases ranging from four—to 20-fold. Based on six unpublished industry studies, FDA admitted that IGF-1 levels in rBGH milk were consistently and statistically increased, and that these were further increased by pasteurization; these increases were also admitted by others. Included among these is one by Lilly Industries, in its application for marketing authorization to the European Community Committee for Veterinary Products, admitting that rBGH milk may contain more than 10-fold increase in IGF-1 levels. It should also be noted that pasteurization increases IGF-1 levels by a further 70%, presumably by disrupting protein binding, and since standard analytic techniques for IGF-1 in rBGH milk may underestimate its levels by up to 40-fold.

4. *IGF-1 Is Readily Absorbed from the Intestine into the Blood*

Contrary to Section 2 of FDA's 6/8/2000 Docket No. 98P-1194 response to the December 5, 1998 Citizen Petition of the Center for Food Safety, IGF-1 is a peptide and not a protein, and as such is readily absorbed into the blood. Even more compelling is evidence of marked growth promoting effects following short-term feeding tests in rats. FDA's Section 2 thus reflects a misunderstanding relating to "the possibility of IGF-1 surviving digestion."

5. *Increased IGF-1 Levels Increase Risks of Breast, Colon and Prostate Cancers*

Thus, increased levels of IGF-1 have been shown to increase risks of breast cancer by up to seven-fold in 19 publications, risks of colon cancer in 10 publications, and prostate cancer in 7 publications.

6. *Increased IGF-1 Levels Inhibit Apoptosis*

Of generally unrecognized, critical importance is the fact that increased IGF-1 levels block natural defense mechanisms against the growth and development of early submicroscopic cancers, known as apoptosis or programmed self destruction.

7. *Bovine Growth Hormone Increases Twinning Rates*

As increased rate of twinning in cows injected with rBGH was admitted by Monsanto on its November 1993 Posilac label. rBGH increases ovulation and embryo survival, and increases the incidence of fraternal twins. "Because multiple gestations are more prone to complications such as premature delivery, congenital defects and pregnancy-induced hypertension in the mother than singleton pregnancies, the finding s of this study suggest that women contemplating pregnancy might consider substituting meat and dairy products with other protein sources, especially in countries that allow growth hormone administration to cattle."

8. *The International Ban on the Use and Imports of rBGH Dairy Products*

Based on the veterinary and public health concerns detailed in this Petition, the use and import of rBGH dairy products has been banned by Canada, 29 European nations, Norway, Switzerland, Japan, New Zealand, and Australia.

It should further be noted that on June 30, 1999, the Codex Alimentarius Commission, the United Nations Food Safety Agency representing 101 nations worldwide, ruled unanimously not to endorse or set a safety standard for rBGH milk.

9. *The FDA Policy on Labeling rBGH Milk*

The FDA has misled dairy producers and consumers with regard to its requirement for labeling of rBGH milk, to the effect that "No significant difference has been shown between milk derived from rBST-treated and non-rBST treated cows." This, however, is misleading in extreme as the "FDA has determined it lacks the basis for requiring such labeling in its statute." This was admitted in a 7/27/94 letter by Jerold R. Mande, Executive Director to the FDA Commissioner, to Harold Rudnick, State of New York Department of Agriculture and Markets.

C. CLAIM FOR CATEGORICAL EXCLUSION

A claim for categorical exclusion is asserted pursuant to 21 CFR 25.24 (a)11.

D. CERTIFICATION

The undersigned certify, that, to their best knowledge and belief, this petition includes all information and views on which the petition relies, and also that it includes representative data and information known to the petitioner which are unfavorable to the petition.

This petition, supported by 61 scientific references, was ignored by the FDA.

Samuel S. Epstein, M.D.
Chairman, Cancer Prevention Coalition
Professor emeritus Occupational and Environmental Medicine
University of Illinois at Chicago

Ronnie Cummins
Executive Director
Organic Consumers Association

John Kinsman
President
Family Farm Defenders

Arpad Pusztai, Ph.D., FRSE

Jeffrey Smith
Executive Director
Institute for Responsible Technology

IMMINENT HEALTH HAZARD FROM HORMONAL MEAT

January 29, 2010

Kathleen Sebelius
Secretary of Health and Human Services
U.S. Department of Health and Human Services

Margaret Hamburg, M.D.
Commissioner of Food and Drugs

Citizen Petition
Dockets Management Branch
Office of Management
5630 Fishers Lane, Room 1061
Rockville, MD 20852

CC: Congressman John Conyers
CC: Congressman Dennis Kucinich

    The undersigned submits this petition on behalf of the Cancer Prevention Coalition, Samuel S. Epstein, M.D., Chairman; Massachusetts Institute of Technology, Nicholas Ashford, Ph.D., J.D., Professor of Technology and Policies; Organic Consumers Association, Ronnie Cummins, Executive Director; and Health and Medicine Policy Research Group, Quentin D. Young, M.D., Chairman.
    Based on a review of the scientific literature, Food and Drug Administration (FDA) Freedom of Information Summaries, other U.S. Government reports, and World Health Organization (WHO) reports, we conclude that the use of natural and synthetic anabolics in meat production poses serious carcinogenic and other hazards to consumers, with particular reference to breast and other reproductive cancers. For these reasons, we petition the federal government to:

- Recognize these hazards as "imminent hazards" for the purpose of appropriate regulatory action to eliminate their use and likely human exposure.

This Petition is based on the following evidence:

1. *The Carcinogenicity of Natural Anabolics*

   a. *Estradiol-17B*

   Based on an exhaustive review of the scientific literature, the International Agency for Research on Cancer (IARC) confirmed the carcinogenicity of estradiol in experimental animals, inducing mammary, testicular, other reproductive tumors, and tumors at other sites, and concluded that it was of comparable potency to diethylstilbestrol, an illegal synthetic anabolic. IARC subsequently concluded that the evidence of estradiol's carcinogenicity to animals was "sufficient", and that it was "causally associated" with reproductive cancers in women.

   b. *Testosterone*

   On the basis of a review of the scientific literature, testosterone was classified by IARC as a Group 2A carcinogen. IARC concluded that the evidence of its carcinogenicity in rodents was "sufficient," and that it "may be involved in the genesis of (prostatitis) tumors in humans." These carcinogenic effects have also been recognized by WHO. Following administration of testosterone to rodents, "the incidence of prostatic tumors was higher than in control animals (and the incidence of uterine tumors was surprisingly high."

   c. *Progesterone*

   On the basis of a review of the scientific literature, IARC concluded that the evidence for its carcinogenicity, based on the induction of mammary, ovarian and uterine cancers in rodents, was "sufficient."

   d. *Enhanced infant sensitivity*

   There is substantial literature on the enhanced carcinogenic sensitivity of neonatal rodents to natural anabolics, both individually and in combination, and to synthetic anabolics, such as diethylstilbestrol. Illustratively, "neonatal exposure of mice to progesterone plus estradiol-17B resulted in an increased incidence of mammary tumors. Furthermore, there is a substantial literature on the increased susceptibility of infant and young rodents and humans to a wide range of carcinogens, including natural anabolics and diethylstilbestrol (DES).

2. *The Carcinogenicity of Synthetic Anabolics*

   a. *Trenbolone Acetate*

   There are no published data on the carcinogenicity of Trenbolone, a synthetic steroid resembling testosterone. However, unpublished and inadequately documented industry data have demonstrated its carcinogenicity to mice and rates. These findings include: "Significant increases in hepatic proliferative lesions (neoplasia and hyperplasia) in male and female (mice)—and in increased incidence of pancreatic islet tumors" in rats. These carcinogenic effects have also been recognized by WHO. However, these conclusions were dismissed by FDA "on the basis of direct and ancillary evidence."

   b. *Zeranol*

   There are no published data on the carcinogenicity of Zeranol, a non-steroidal synthetic estrogen. However, unpublished and inadequately documented industry data have demonstrated the "induction of anterior lobe pituitary adenomas" in male rats. These carcinogenic effects have also been recognized by WHO.

   c. *Melengesterol Acetate (MGA)*

   There are no published data on the carcinogenicity of MGA, a synthetic progestin. A 1966 Food Additive Petition to the FDA, summarizing the toxicology of MGA and on the basis of which its use was approved, omitted any reference to carcinogenicity. However, an internal industry report documented the induction of a statistically significant incidence of mammary tumors in female mice; these results were subsequently published.

3. *Residues of Anabolics Following Legal Administration for Meat Production*

   The legal route for administration of natural anabolics and of synthetic anabolics, other than MGA, is subcutaneous implantation of pellets in the ear. In October 1989, FDA approved the re-implantation of steers with estradiol benzoate and progesterone (Synovex-S) in the mid-point of their feeing period. There has been no requirement for any pre-slaughter withdrawal period for over three decades.

Both USDA and FDA have assured the public that meat products are routinely monitored for residues of animal drugs and other industrial chemicals through offensive statements:

- "Since 1987, USDA and FDA have been monitoring volatile levels of residues of animal drugs, pesticides, and industrial chemicals in food animals."
- "The program has expanded greatly since its inception, and because the use of many pesticides has declined, a greater emphasis is now placed on testing for animal drugs."
- "The program is designed to ensure that the compounds most likely to be present in food animals are included in the nationwide monitoring residue plan. The program has the flexibility to keep up with current usage of animal drugs."
- "Samples of meat and poultry products are collected from healthy appearing animals at domestic slaughter establishments using a statistically based, random sampling plan."
- "Surveillance programs are designed to distinguish those areas of the livestock and poultry populations in which residue problems exist, to measure the extent of the problems, and to evaluate the impact of actions initiated to reduce the occurrence of residues."
- "FSIS (Food Safety and Inspection Service of USDA) collects samples for testing when a problem with residues is suspected."
- "Most residue monitoring program has been supported by an education program targeted at food animal producers, and its success has assisted in the decline of residue violators."
- "The residue monitoring program has been supported by an education program targeted at food animal producers, and its success has assisted in the decline of residue violators."
- "In 1993, approximately one-fourth of one percent of animals tested showed positive for residue violation. In other words, almost 99.74 percent of animals tested showed no residue violations."

However, in contrast to these highly misleading published assurances, FSIS 1993 data indicate that none of approximately 120 million head of livestock slaughtered annually have been monitored for any residues of natural or synthetic anabolics.

The only available residue data are provided in "New Animal Drug Application" (NADA) petitions to FDA, by pharmaceutical companies, manufacturing and formulating the anabolic drugs, as detailed in Freedom of Information Summaries obtained from the FDA. Residue levels were determined by specialized techniques, radio-immune assays, which are not practical for routine monitoring. Despite the requirement of Section 512 of The 1968 Animal Drug Amendments to the Federal Food Inspection Act which stipulates that a manufacturer submitting a NADA must provide "a description of practical methods" for analysis and monitoring of carcinogenic residues in food, no such methods were available in 1973; over two decades later, none are still available. FDA, however, has circumvented this legislative mandate by claiming that "a regulatory method is not needed for the assurance of safety of the approved use of (anabolic) implants because the maximum increased exposure, even considering probable misuse of the drug, is demonstrated to be far below those concentrations considered unsafe."

a. *Estradiol*

Following implantation of steers with Synovex-S (estradiol benzoate and progesterone), estradiol residues in liver, kidney, muscle and fat at 15 days were increased over normal background levels by 6, 9, 12 and 23-fold, respectively; the average residue in fat of untreated controls was 1.8ppt (ng/kg). However, minimizing these data, WHO claimed that estradiol implants "—may produce two-fold to five-fold increases in residue levels and that these fall within the normal range found in untreated bovine animals—", the comparability of which was, however, unspecified.

b. *Testosterone*

Following implantation of heifers with Synovex-H (estradiol benzoate and testosterone propionate), testosterone residues in kidney, liver, muscle and fat at 30 days were increased over normal background levels by 2, 3, 5 and 30-fold, respectively; the average fat level in untreated animals was 26ppt (ng/kg). Similar increased residues have been reported by WHO.

c. *Trenbolone*

Following implantation of heifers with Revalor (Trenbolone acetate and estradiol), the total average residues in beef liver were 50 ppb (µg/kg) at 30 days, while "residues in muscle, kidney and fat were much lower." In contrast to these data, WHO, however, claimed that the 50ppb liver residues were the "highest mean concentrations."

d. *Zeranol*

Following implantation of Ralgro (Zeranol) in steers and heifers, total average residues in muscle, fat, kidney and liver at 15 days were 0.1, 0.3, 1.7, and 8.2ppb. Similar residues have been reported by WHO.

e. *Melengesterol Acetate (MGA)*

Following feeding heifers with MGA, 139 of 174 fat samples contained residues below 10ppb, while the remainder had residues ranging from 10-19ppb at 12 to 24 hours after the last feeding; the sensitivity level of this assay was only 10ppb. It should be noted that WHO has still failed to evaluate the use of MGA; this is in contrast to the requirement that it evaluates all veterinary drugs regulated in at least one country.

4. *Residues of Anabolics Following Illegal Administration*

No data are available on the much higher local and distant residue levels anticipated following intramuscular implantation or injection. A 1986 USDA survey revealed that as many as half the cattle in 32 large feedlots had "misplaced implants." FDA's response was limited in extreme: "part of the carcass containing pellets should continue to be condemned". Such action ignores the probability of high residues in distant organs and tissues due to the anticipated increased absorption of anabolics from highly vascular muscle in contrast to relatively avascular subcutaneous ear tissue. Furthermore, visual inspection and random monitoring could not reveal evidence of intramuscular injection, as opposed to implantation.

5. *Public Health Hazards from Residues of Natural Anabolics in Meat Products*

FDA has consistently dismissed concerns on hazards of natural anabolics in meat:

> "No harmful effects will occur in individuals chronically ingesting animal tissues that contain an incremental increase of endogenous steroid equal to 1% or less of the amount produced daily by the segment of the population with the lowest daily production rate. In the case of Estradiol, prepubertal boys synthesize the least; in the case of testosterone, prepubertal girls synthesize the least. The calculated incremental increase permitted in beef muscle above the amount naturally present in untreated animals are 120ppt

for Estradiol and 0.64ppb for Testosterone. Based upon relative consumption of other tissues versus muscle, safe incremental levels of 480ppt and 2.6ppb for Estradiol and Testosterone, respectively, are established for fat, 360ppt and 1.9ppb for kidney, and 240ppt and 1.3ppb for liver."

"When the sponsor can demonstrate with a suitable assay that under the proposed conditions of use the concentration of residue of the endogenous sex steroid in treated food-producing animals is such that the actual increase in exposure of people will not exceed the permitted increase, then the compound is shown to be safe."

These assurances of safety are flawed for reasons including the following:

a. Consumption of meat products with incremental residues of a specific exogenous anabolic not only increases normal body hormonal levels, but also disturbs complex patters of normal hormonal interaction and balances. Such imbalances pose carcinogenic hazards.
b. The amount of endogenous steroids "produced by the segment of the population with the lowest daily production rate" are infants and young, rather than prepubertal children; daily estradiol production for prepubertal boys, 6.5 µg, is over 50-fold in excess of levels for children under 8, based on IARC data (1, p.42-46). This is of particular significance in view of the enhanced sensitivity of infants to the carcinogenic effects of estrogens (see Section 1d).
c. In the absence of routine monitoring, there is no assurance that "the proposed conditions of use" of the anabolics corresponds to routine feedlot practice. There is in fact evidence to the contrary, resulting in unmonitored residue levels well in excess of those anticipated by FDA (see Section 3).
d. FDA assurances are based on the alleged absence of "harmful effects" of individual anabolics. However, in practice, most implants contain two natural anabolics or one natural and one synthetic anabolic thus invalidating FDA's calculated assumptions. Furthermore, the probability of additive, let alone synergistic hormonal effects has apparently not been considered by FDA (see Section 1d). Of related concern is recent evidence that two xenobiotic pesticides induce synergistic estrogenic effects some 1000-fold greater than those resulting from individual exposures.
e. FDA has failed to consider incremental, additive or synergistic, carcinogenic and estrogenic effects of anabolic steroids together

with those of xenoestrogenic pesticides and other industrial chemical contaminants in meat products.
   f. FDA has failed to recognize the long standing evidence of the approximately 10,000-fold higher potency of estradiol than xenoestrogenic pesticides whose feminizing hazards are of increasing public health concern; such hazards may also include reduction in human male fertility.

6. *Therapeutic Administration of Anabolics*

The therapeutic uses of anabolics do not pose public health hazards. Such uses are extremely limited, compared to large-scale routine feedlot use, and are prescribed by qualified veterinarians, in contrast to feedlot operators. Furthermore, determination of therapeutic effectiveness necessitates pre-slaughter withdrawal.

7. *Public Health Hazards from Residues of Synthetic Anabolics in Meat Products*

The hazards of synthetic anabolics have been trivialized or dismissed by both FDA and WHO:

> "Safe concentrations" or tolerances have been established by FDA for residues of Trenbolone in spite of explicit industry data on its carcinogenicity (see Section 2a); these tolerances range from 50-20ppb for different organs and tissues. Similarly, WHO has established "maximum residue levels" (MRL) based on "Acceptable Daily Intakes" (ADI) for meat and dairy products.

> "Safe concentrations" for total Zeranol residues have also been established by FDA, in spite of explicit industry carcinogenicity data, recognized by WHO, and the carcinogenicity of its metabolite Zearalenone (see Section 2b). Similarly, WHO have established ADI-based "Acceptable Residue Levels."

FDA has established a tolerance "in edible tissues" for MGA in spite of explicit industry carcinogenicity data (see Section 2c). WHO has failed to evaluate MGA in spite of its use in the U.S. for nearly three decades.

The public health hazards of synthetic anabolics are in general comparable to those of natural anabolics. Of particular concern, however, are the much higher residues of synthetic (in the ppb range), than the natural anabolics (in the ppt range). The concepts of tolerances, ADI and MRL are inappropriate in extreme for any carcinogen, let alone for high residues of carcinogens deliberately introduced into the food supply.

There is substantial evidence challenging the validity of classifying carcinogens as epigenetic, on the basis of bacterial gene mutation tests, for which thresholds or Acceptable Daily Intake (ADI) levels are claimed, as genotoxic. It should be emphasized that asbestos, benzene, arsenic and non-steroidal and steroidal estrogens, all IARC recognized potent Group 1 carcinogens, are inactive in bacterial tests and hence classified as epigenetic, However, they are all mutagenic and thus genotoxic in mammalian systems. Apart from this, hormonal anabolics are mutagenic in mammalian test systems and are thus genotoxic (Tables 1 and 2). There is also substantial scientific evidence challenging the existence of thresholds for any carcinogen. This evidence is even more persuasive for exposures involving unpredictable synergistic interactions. There is no scientific basis for WHO claims that ADI levels can be set for natural and synthetic anabolic carcinogens, or for claims that ADI levels can be based on "no-hormonal-effect levels" of synthetic anabolic carcinogens.

8. *Misleading Assurances of Safety by U.S. Regulatory Agencies and "Expert Committees"*

The repeated misleading assurances by USDA and FDA since 1979 on the safety of natural and synthetic anabolics are consistent with a similar prior record with regard to DES, including suppression of residue data. Compounding these concerns is longstanding evidence of conflicts of interest in senior agency personnel and their consultants.

As clearly evidenced in a series of General Accounting Office investigations and Congressional hearings, USDA inspection and FDA registration and residue-tolerance programs are in near total disarray. A 1986 report, "Human Food Safety and Regulation of Animal Drugs," unanimously approved by the House Committee on Government Operations, concluded that the "FDA has consistently disregarded its responsibility—has repeatedly put what it perceives are interests of veterinarians and the livestock industry ahead of its legal obligation to protect consumers—jeopardizing the health and safety of consumers meat, milk, and poultry." These criticisms appear equally appropriate today. Illustratively, in response on questions on hormonal meat raised in February 1996 by the European Commission Washington Delegation, the USDA responded with assurances that less than 0.25% of animals tested annually proved positive for "residue violations." In fact, however, no cattle have been monitored for sex hormones.

Similar concerns relate to exculpatory reports by Joint WHO Expert Committees on Food Additives. The membership of these committees reflects disproportionate representation of U.S. senior regulatory officials and of veterinary and food scientists, with minimal if any involvement of independent experts in preventive medicine, public health and carcinogenesis. The European Commission Scientific Conference of November 29-December 1, 1995 also reflects such imbalanced representation. While Conference participate of "scientists directly employed" by industry was "generally refused," no apparent attempt was made to identify or exclude industry consultants, contractees or grantees. Furthermore, the Conference based its finding and conclusions largely on unpublished industry data. As admitted by Steering Committee member Dr. F. W. Kenny, "all assessment data are provided by companies and this implies a regulatory gap," particularly in view of the confidentially of these data; industry is "capable of giving good results, but they will not necessarily always do so." Similar constraints in data generated and interpreted by industry and their consultants have been well documented.

9. *Conclusions*

Some three decades ago, Roy Hertz, then director of endocrinology of the National Cancer Institute and world authority on hormonal cancer, warned of the carcinogenic risks of estrogenic feed additives, particularly for hormonally sensitive tissues such as breast tissue, because they could increase normal body hormonal levels and disturb delicately poised hormonal balances. Hertz pointed to evidence from innumerable animal tests and human clinical experience that such imbalance can be carcinogenic. Hertz also warned of the essentially uncontrolled and unregulated use of these extremely potent biological agents, no dietary levels of which can be regarded as safe. These warnings are even more apt today.

Lifelong exposure to hormonal anabolics poses significant carcinogenic risks, particularly for breast and other reproductive cancers, whose rates have sharply escalated over recent decades. Such exposures may also pose serious feminizing risks.

TABLE 1: CARCINOGENICITY AND GENOTOXICITY OF HORMONAL ANABOLICS*

ANABOLIC	CARCINOGENICITY	MAMMALIAN GENOTOXICITY
ESTRADIOL-17B	+	+
TESTOSTERONE	+	+
PROGESTERONE	+	+
TRENBOLONE-17B	+	+
ZERANOL	+	-
MELENGESTEROL	+	No Data Available

TABLE 2: GENOTOXICITY OF HORMONAL ANABOLICS*

ANABOLIC	GENOTOXIC TEST SYSTEM
ESTRADIOL-17B	Aneuploidy, aberrant nucleotides and UDS rodent cells in vitro Micronuclei human cells in vitro Transformation, and DNA adducts by metabolites Chromosome aberrations by metabolites in vitro
TESTOSTERONE	As for estradiol in view of in vivo aromatization Transformation hamster cells in vitro
PROGESTERONE	Chromosome aberrations human cells in vitro Chromosome aberrations dog and hamster meiotic cells in vivo
TRENBOLONE-17B	Micronuclei and transformation hamster cells by metabolites in vitro
ZERANOL	Positive Rec-assay B, subtilis
ZEARALENONE	Positive Rec-assay B. subtilis Chromosome aberrations hamster cells in vitro DNA adducts in mice in vivo

This petition is submitted by:

Samuel S. Epstein, M.D.
Chairman, Cancer Prevention Coalition
Professor emeritus Occupational and Environmental Medicine
University of Illinois at Chicago

Nicholas Ashford, Ph.D., J.D.
Professor of Technology and Policy
Massachusetts Institute of Technology

Ronnie Cummins
Executive Director, Organic Consumers Association

Quentin D. Young, M.D.
Chairman, Health & Medicine Policy Research Group
Past President, American Public Health Association

PRESS RELEASES & HUFFINGTON POST BLOGS, 1995-2011

January 15, 1995	Lice Won't Kill You but Its Treatment Can: Experts Call for Ban on Lindane Shampoos
January 25, 1995	"Research Cures Cancer" Campaign Misleads Public and Congress
February 22, 1998	Major Cosmetic and Toiletry Ingredient Poses Avoidable Cancer Risks, Warns Professor of Environmental Medicine at University of Illinois School Of Public Health
January 7, 2000	New Initiatives in Personal Care Product Safety
February 7, 2000	Perfume: Cupid's Arrow or Poison Dart
January 15, 2001	Undisclosed Carcinogens in Cosmetics and Personal Care Products Pose Avoidable Risks Of Cancer
April 8, 2001	Administration Proposal to Serve Irradiated Beef to School Children Poses Cancer, Genetic and Other Risks
June 12, 2001	The American Cancer Society Is Threatening the National Cancer Program
October 10, 2001	American Academy of Pediatrics Guidelines for Treating Behavioral Disorders in Children with Ritalin Ignores Evidence of Cancer Risks
May 9, 2002	Escalating Incidence of Childhood Cancer Remains Ignored by the National Cancer Institute
July 11, 2002	Phthalates in Cosmetics Are Suspect, But Carcinogens Even More So

August 15, 2002	Groups Call For Labeling of Cosmetics and Toiletries, Citing Cancer and Other Health Risks
November 1, 2002	USDA's Allowing Schools to Serve Irradiated Meat Is Reckless
May 8, 2003	Public Remains Uninformed of Escalating Incidence of Childhood Cancer and Its Avoidable Causes
May 23, 2003	The American Cancer Society Misleads The Public in the May 26 Discovery Health Channel Program
February 23, 2004	Spinning the Losing Cancer War
July 1, 2004	Environmental Working Group Report on Personal Care Products: Ambitious, But Flawed
August 6, 2004	High Time to Label Fragrance Allergens
October 14, 2004	Europe Leads the Way in Cosmetic Product Safety
February 28, 2005	Time To Protect Babies from Dangerous Products
April 10, 2006	National School Lunches: Unsafe At Any Eating
December 16, 2009	Reckless Indifference of the American Cancer Society to Cancer Prevention
January 26, 2010	President Obama and the Congress Must Take Action on Cancer Prevention
March 29, 2010	Frank Conflicts of Interest in the National Cancer Institute
May 4, 2010	Cancer Prevention Coalition Urged Support of the Safe Chemicals Act
May 7, 2010	Protect Children's Health from Bisphenol-A
January 4, 2011	Unrecognized Dangers of Formaldehyde
January 24, 2011	Danger of Bone Cancer from Fluoride in Toothpaste, and Drinking Water
November 18, 2011	The American Cancer Society Ignores Evidence On Avoidable Causes Of Childhood Cancers
December 15, 2011	Multiple Carcinogens in Johnson & Johnson's Baby Shampoo

January 15, 1995

LICE WON'T KILL YOU BUT ITS TREATMENT CAN

Experts Call For Ban On Lindane Shampoos

According to scientific experts, commonly prescribed lice shampoos can cause fatal childhood cancer. The Cancer Prevention Coalition (CPC) will inform the public of this danger at a press briefing on January 17, 1995 at 12 noon.

About six million Americans, mainly children, are infested with lice each year. A common treatment for lice is a shampoo containing the pesticide lindane. Recent epidemiological studies have reported high rates of brain cancer in children treated with lindane shampoos. These findings are significant in light of the dramatic 38% increase of childhood brain and nervous system cancer rates from 1973 to 1991.

Additional evidence comes from recent studies linking lindane exposure to increased risks of non-Hodgkin's lymphoma, and also from long-standing evidence on fatal blood diseases including aplastic anemia and leukemia. These findings are supported by experimental evidence of carcinogenicity confirmed by the World Health Organization, the Environmental protection Agency, and the Department of health and Human Services; on the basis of such hazards, the EPA and several other countries have restricted lindane's use in agriculture, and other countries have banned it. Additionally, lindane is a known neurotoxin—resulting in seizures and brain damages at dose levels used in the shampoos.

CPC has sent letters to the Chicago Board, and to other local and state authorities urging that they warn parents of the dangers of lindane shampoo and to encourage them to seek out safer treatments. CPC has also filed a citizen petition with the Food and Drug Administration calling for a ban of lindane-based shampoos.

Speakers at the press conference will include Chair Dr. Samuel Epstein, CPC Board members Dr. Quentin Young and Dr. Peter Orris, parent Community Council President Mr. James Deanes, and Legal Director of the New York-based Center for Constitutional Rights, Michael Deutsch. The speakers will discuss the public health implications of these data and will offer information about safer alternatives.

Commenting on the widely-prescribed use of lindane, Dr. Quentin Young, CPC Board member said, "It is a serious medical tragedy when these products are used with such good intentions and can have such tragic outcomes."

ENDORSER:

Michael Deutsch, Legal Director, Center for Constitutional Rights

January 25, 1995

CANCER RESEARCH CAMPAIGN MISLEADS PUBLIC AND CONGRESS

A statement by national organizations representing over 5 million Americans warned of misleading efforts by "treatment groups" and the cancer drug industry to allocate more tax dollars towards funding cancer research.

The statement responded to a Washington, D.C. kick-off of the National Coalition for Cancer Research's industry-sponsored "Research Cures Cancer" campaign, which is lobbying Congress to increase support for the National Cancer Institute's (NCI) programs.

The statement sent a message to policymakers that further funding is not going to cure cancer. It stressed that NCI's priorities are fixated on research on treatment and molecular biology, while issues of environmental and workplace-induced cancers are trivialized. The reason for the failed war against cancer is not a shortage of funds but their gross misallocation. NCI has devoted minimal funding to cancer prevention. Furthermore, NCI has failed to inform Congress and the public of a wide range of avoidable causes of environmental and occupational cancers.

The organizations concluded by calling for an appointment of a new director at NCI who is more responsive to growing national concerns on prevention of the cancer epidemic.

Cancer Research Campaign Misleads the Public and Congress

On January 25, 1995 in Washington, D.C., the National Coalition for Cancer Research will launch an industry-funded "Research Cures Cancer" campaign which misled Congress and the public into the groundless belief that further research is the answer to the cancer epidemic. The Coalition, sponsored by the American Cancer Society and the cancer drug industry, is lobbying Congress and taxpayers to provide the National Cancer Institute (NCI) with more research funding.

Twenty-five years since President Nixon and Congress inaugurated the National Cancer Act, the war against cancer has failed. In spite of over $25 billion of taxpayers funding, cancer rates have escalated to epidemic proportions while our ability to treat and cure most cancers remains largely unchanged.

For decades, NCI policy and priorities have remained narrowly fixated on research on treatment and basic molecular biology. Despite its questionable relevance, molecular biology receives over 50% of NCI's $2 billion annual budget. Nevertheless, molecular biologist and current director of the National Institutes of Health, Dr. Harold Varmus, is encouraging still more emphasis on basic molecular biology research in the NCI.

The reason for the failed war against cancer is not a shortage of funds but their gross misallocation. NCI has directed a minimal priority to cancer prevention. Furthermore, NCI has failed to inform Congress and the public of a wide range of avoidable carcinogens in the air, water, food, consumer products and the workplace. Research on such exposures receives a miniscule 5% of NCI's annual budget. Reduction of exposures to carcinogens in the workplace and the environment are likely to reverse the current epidemic.

With the NCI directorship being vacated next month, it is time to see the NCI face up to escalating cancer rates and its imbalanced preoccupation with research on treatment and molecular biology. As organizations representing 5 million Americans, we demand that President Clinton appoint a leading scientist with a strong credentials and clear commitment to cancer prevention as director of the NCI.

The Cancer Prevention Coalition and the co-signing organizations also demand that:

- NCI must be held accountable for its failed policies and the $25 billion in taxpayer support in the war against cancer.
- NCI must undergo radical reforms in its programs, priorities, and leadership.
- Cancer prevention must receive greater emphasis in NCI policies.
- The NCI budget must be held hostage to such reforms under the terms of the Government Performance and Results Act of 1993.

CO-SIGNING ORGANIZATIONS:

Breast Cancer Action
San Francisco, CA

Cancer Prevention Coalition
Chicago, IL

Center for Constitutional Rights
New York, NY

Center for Media & Democracy
Madison, WI

Citizen Action
Washington, DC

Environmental Research Foundation
Annapolis, MD

Food and Water, Inc.
Marshfield, VT

Greenpeace USA
Chicago, IL

Mother Jones Magazine
San Francisco, CA

Pesticide Action Network
San Francisco, CA

Project Impact
Oakland, CA

Pure Food Campaign
Washington, DC

Radiation and Public Health Project
New York, NY

Women's Community Cancer Project
Boston, MA

Women's Environment & Development Organization
New York, NY

February 22, 1998

MAJOR COSMETIC AND TOILETRY INGREDIENT POSES AVOIDABLE CANCER RISKS, WARNS PROFESSOR OF ENVIRONMENTAL MEDICINE AT UNIVERSITY OF ILLINOIS SCHOOL OF PUBLIC HEALTH

As reported on CBS Morning News today, the National Toxicology Program (NTP) recently found that repeated skin application to mouse skin of diethanolamine (DEA), or its fatty acid derivative cocamide-DEA, induced liver and kidney cancer. Besides this "clear evidence of carcinogenicity," NTP also emphasized that DEA is readily absorbed through the skin and accumulates in organs, such as the brain, where it induces chronic toxic effects.

High concentrations of DEA-based detergents are commonly used in a wide range of cosmetics and toiletries, including shampoos, hair dyes and conditioners, lotions, creams and bubble baths, besides liquid dishwashing and laundry soaps. Lifelong use of these products thus clearly poses major avoidable cancer risks to the great majority of U.S. consumers, particularly infants and young children.

Further increasing these cancer risks is longstanding evidence that DEA readily interacts with nitrite preservatives or contaminants in cosmetics or toiletries to form nitrosodiethanolamine (NDELA), another carcinogen as well recognized by Federal agencies and institutions and the World Health Organization, which, like DEA, is also rapidly absorbed through the skin. In 1979, FDA warned that over 40% of all cosmetic products were contaminated with NDELA and called for industry "to take immediate action to eliminate this carcinogen from cosmetic products." In two 1991 surveys, 27 out of 29 products were found to be contaminated with high concentrations of this carcinogen, results which were subsequently confirmed by the FDA. Based on this information, the European Union and European industry have both taken strong action to reduce or eliminate DEA and NDELA from cosmetics and toiletries. In sharp contrast, the FDA has taken no such action, nor has it responded to a 1996 petition from the Cancer Prevention Coalition to phase out the use of DEA or to label DEA-containing products with an explicit cancer warning. The mainstream U.S. industry has been similarly unresponsive, even to the extent of ignoring an explicit warning by the Cosmetics, Toiletries and Fragrance Association to discontinue uses of DEA. Such reckless intransigence is in strong contrast to the responsiveness of the growing safe cosmetic industry.

Tom Mower, CEO of Neways Inc., a major distributor of carcinogen-free cosmetics, emphasizes: "I see no reason at all to use DEA, as there are safe and cost-effective alternatives which we have been using in a wide range of our cosmetics and toiletries for the last decade."

Faced with escalating cancer rates, now striking more than one in three Americans, FDA should take immediate action to prevent further exposure to the avoidable carcinogens DEA and NDELA in cosmetics, toiletries and liquid soaps. Safe and effective alternatives to DEA are readily available.

January 7, 2000

NEW INITIATIVES IN PERSONAL CARE PRODUCT SAFETY

Fragrances and Perfumes

As emphasized in the Safe Shopper's Bible, fragrances and perfumes in mainstream cosmetics and toiletries, besides in soaps and other household products, are leading causes of allergy, sensitization, and irritation. Their toxicity is also in serious question as is their contribution to indoor air pollution.

The National Institute of Occupational Safety and Health has reported that the fragrance industry uses up to 3,000 ingredients, predominantly synthetic, some 900 of which were identified as toxic. However, the industry is not required to disclose ingredients of fragrances and perfumes on their labels due to trade secrecy considerations. The FDA supports this non-disclosure on the grounds that "consumers are not adversely affected—and should not be deprived of the enjoyment" of these products.

An analysis of six different mainstream perfumes by Scientific Instrument Services, released in November 1998, identified over 800 ingredients with distinctive patterns for each perfume. These ingredients include a wide range of volatile and semi-volatile organic chemicals, which are thus significant contributors to indoor pollution.

On May 11, 1999, the California Environmental Health Network filed a Citizen Petition with the FDA requiring warning labels on all fragrances which are marketed without prior adequate safety testing. Additionally, the petition requested the FDA to take administrative action and declare Calvin Klein's "Eternity eau de parfum" as "misbranded." This petition has been supported and endorsed by the CPC. While Eternity perfume was based on recent analysis of the perfume by two independent laboratories, Scientific Instrument Services and the cosmetic industry's Research Institute of Fragrance Materials Laboratory. Of all 41 ingredients identified, no toxicity data are available on some, data on most are inadequate, and others are known to be toxic to the skin, mucous membranes, respiratory tract, and reproductive and nervous system by routes including skin absorption and inhalation. Additionally, two ingredients (phenylmethyl acetic acid ester and 2,6-bis (1,1-dimethylethyl)-4-methyl-phenol) were identified as carcinogens. The FDA has 180 days to respond to this petition. However, any positive response is most unlikely.

Neways International, a leading alternative safe consumer products company, has taken a precedential initiative in the area of fragrance safety.

The few fragrances used in Neways personal care products contain less than 10 ingredients, most of which are natural. As importantly, none of the few synthetics used are known to be toxic or carcinogenic. In the near future, these products will be labeled accordingly.

Surfactants:

A wide range of personal care products including shampoos, hair conditions, cleansers, lotions, and creams, besides household products such as soaps and cleaning products, contain surfactants or detergents such as ethoxylated alcohols, polysorbates, and laureths. These ingredients are generally contaminated with high concentrations of the highly volatile 1,4-dioxane, which is both readily inhaled and absorbed through the skin. The carcinogenicity of dioxane in rodents was first reported in 1965 and subsequently confirmed in other studies including by the National Cancer Institute in 1978; the predominant sites of cancer were nasal passages in rats and liver in mice. Epidemiological studies on dioxane-exposed furniture makers have reported suggestive evidence of excess nasal passage cancers. On the basis of such evidence, the Consumer Product Safety Commission concluded, "the presence of 1,4-dioxane, even as a trace contaminant, is a cause of concern." These avoidable risks of cancer in numerous personal care, besides other consumer products, is inexcusable, particularly as the dioxane is readily removed from surfactants during their manufacture by a process known as "vacuum stripping."

Again, Neways now stands alone in certifying and labeling the surfactants in its personal care products as "dioxane-free," and thus sets an important precedent to the entire personal care products industry.

February 7, 2000

PERFUME: CUPID'S ARROW OR POISON DART

Lovers looking for the perfect Valentine's gift should think twice before giving a bottle of toxic chemicals to their sweethearts. Recent analysis of Calvin Klein's "Eternity Eau de Parfum" (Eternity) by an industry laboratory specializing in fragrance chemistry revealed 41 ingredients. These include some known to be toxic to the skin, respiratory tract, nervous, and reproductive systems, and others known to be carcinogens; no toxicity data are available on several ingredients, while data on most are inadequate. Additionally, some ingredients are volatile and a source of indoor air pollution. Since 1995, several consumers have complained to the Food and Drug Administration (FDA) of neurological and respiratory problems due to Eternity.

The analysis was recently commissioned by the Environmental Health Network (EHN) as many members had complained of asthma, migraine, sensitization, or multiple chemical sensitivity when exposed to Eternity. Based on this analysis, EHN filed a Citizen Petition with the FDA on May 11, 1999, which was subsequently endorsed by the Cancer Prevention Coalition. The petition requests that the FDA take administrative action and declare Eternity "misbranded" or "adulterated" since it does not carry a warning label as required by the terms of the Food, Drug, and Cosmetic Act and the Fair Packaging and Labeling Act. Grounds for requesting the warning label include FDA regulation 21CFR Sec. 740/10: "Each ingredient used in a cosmetic product and each finished cosmetic product shall be adequately substantiated for safety prior to marketing. Any such ingredient or product whose safety is not adequately substantiated prior to marketing is misbranded unless it contains the following conspicuous statement on the principal display panel: Warning: the safety of this product has not been determined."

Since May, over 700 consumers with health problems from exposure to various mainstream fragrances have written to the FDA supporting EHN's petition. The FDA responded on November 30 to the effect that they had been unable to reach a decision on the grounds of "other priorities and the limited availability of resources." The petition is thus still open for further public complaints and endorsements.

A wide range of mainstream fragrances and perfumes, predominantly based on synthetic ingredients, are used in numerous cosmetics and toiletries, and also soaps and other household products. Currently, the fragrance industry is virtually unregulated. Its recklessness is abetted and compounded by FDA's complicity. The FDA has refused to require the industry to disclose ingredients due to trade secrecy considerations, and still takes the position that "consumers are not adversely affected—and should not be deprived of the enjoyment" of these products. The Cancer Prevention Coalition and EHN take the unequivocal position that the FDA should implement its own regulations and act belatedly to protect consumer health and safety.

Valentine sweethearts should switch to organically grown (pesticide-free) roses or other flowers as safe alternatives to mainstream perfumes.

ENDORSER:

Amy Marsh
President of the Environmental Health Network
Larkspur, California

January 15, 2001

UNDISCLOSED CARCINOGENS IN COSMETICS AND PERSONAL CARE PRODUCTS POSE AVOIDABLE RISKS OF CANCER

Government scientists recently identified a group of toxic chemicals known as phthalates in urine of adults, with highest levels in premenopausal women, resulting from inhalation and skin exposure to volatile parent ingredients used extensively as solvents and plasticizers in personal care and cosmetic (PCC) products. These include perfumes, shampoos, hair sprays and nail polishes. These findings raise major concerns in view of documented evidence, dating back to 1985, that these phthalates induce birth defects, low sperm counts, and other reproductive toxicity in experimental animals. The Food and Drug Administration (FDA), authorized by the 1938 Food, Drug and Cosmetics Act to ban unsafe PCC products, responded that it will now "consider" this longstanding information. While obviously important, the phthalate findings merely reflect the tip of an iceberg of more fundamental problems which have received minimal, if any, attention, from Congress, the media and the public.

The FDA's relaxed response reflects reckless regulatory abdication matched by unresponsiveness of mainstream industries. A 1990 report by the U.S. General Accounting Office charging that the FDA commits no resources for assessing PCC safety had no impact on the agency's policies. The agency's sole requirement is restricted to ingredient labeling of PCC products, with the exception of fragrances and perfumes. With rare exceptions, such as children's bubble baths, the FDA has never required industry to label PCC products with any warning of well-documented toxic or cancer risks, nor has it banned the sale of unsafe products to an unsuspecting public.

Black and dark brown permanent hair dyes contain numerous ingredients, such as diaminoanisole and FD&C Red 33, recognized as carcinogens in experimental animals. This evidence is supported by studies establishing that regular use of these dyes poses major risks of relatively rare cancers—non-Hodgkin's lymphoma, Hodgkin's disease and multiple myeloma.

Cosmetic grade talc is carcinogenic in experimental animals. Also, frequent genital dusting with talc, routinely practiced by some 17% of women, increases risks of ovarian cancer.

A group of widely used preservatives, such as quaternium15 and bronopol, widely used in baby products, though not carcinogenic themselves, break down to release formaldehyde, a potent irritant and carcinogen.

Lanolin, widely used on babies' skin and nipples of nursing mothers, is commonly contaminated with DDT and other carcinogenic pesticides.

Commonly used PCC detergents and foaming agents, such as polysorbates and PEG, are usually contaminated with the volatile carcinogen dioxane, although this could be easily removed by vacuum stripping during manufacture.

DEA, another widely used chemical detergent, has been known since 1975 to combine with nitrite preservatives or contaminants in PCC products to form a highly carcinogenic nitrosamine. Furthermore, recent government studies showed that DEA itself is also carcinogenic following application to mouse skin.

Citizen petitions to the FDA by the Cancer Prevention Coalition in 1994 and 1996 detailing evidence on the cancer risks of talc and DEA-containing products, respectively, and "Seeking Carcinogenic Labeling" on these products, met with no substantive response.

Concerns on cancer risks from PCC products are emphasized by: lifelong use of multiple products by the majority of the U.S. population; the ready skin absorption of carcinogenic ingredients, further increased by detergents, especially when left on the skin for prolonged periods; and by decades-long suppression of information by the FDA and industry, abetted by a roll-over media, in flagrant denial of consumers' right-to-know. Mainstream industry products thus pose major risks of avoidable cancer. Their role in the escalating incidence of cancer, now striking one in two men and one in three women in their lifetimes, remains largely unrecognized by our apparently health conscious society. Armed with such information, consumers should protect themselves by shopping for safe alternative products available from the growing non-mainstream industry.

April 8, 2001

ADMINISTRATION PROPOSAL TO SERVE IRRADIATED BEEF TO SCHOOL CHILDREN POSES CANCER, GENETIC AND OTHER RISKS

The recent proposal by the Bush Administration to allow irradiated ground beef into the National School-Lunch Program will endanger the health of tens of millions of school children and should be withdrawn immediately.

"The government's assertion that irradiated food is safe for human consumption does not even pass the laugh test," states Samuel S. Epstein, M.D., emeritus professor of environmental medicine at University of Illinois School of Public Health, Chicago. "Exposing America's school children to the hazards of irradiated food is reckless negligence, compounded by the absence of any warning to parents".

Irradiated meat is a very different product than natural meat. This is hardly surprising as the Food and Drug Administration's (FDA) approved irradiation dosage of 450,000 rads is approximately 150 million times greater than that of a chest x-ray. Apart from high levels of benzene, new chemicals known as "unique radiolytic products" were identified in irradiated meat in U.S. Army tests in 1977 and recognized as carcinogenic. Later tests identified other chemicals shown to induce genetic toxicity. In sharp contrast to FDA's claims of safety, based on grossly inadequate testing which fails to meet the agency's minimal standards and which were explicitly rebutted by its own expert committees, there is well-documented scientific evidence that eating irradiated meat poses grave risks of cancer and genetic damage. Irradiated meat is also highly susceptible to cross-contamination with food poisoning bacteria.

Nevertheless, the meat and irradiation industries, with FDA's complicity, are lobbying aggressively to sanitize the agency's weak labeling requirements for irradiated meat and other food by eliminating the word "irradiated" in favor of "electronic (or cold) pasteurization". This euphemistic absurdity would circumvent consumer's fundamental right-to-know.

Furthermore, irradiation masks grossly unsanitary conditions in slaughterhouses and meat processing plants. Irradiation is thus a major disincentive to decades-long overdue basic sanitary practices essential for the prevention of Salmonella, E.coli O157, and other pathogenic food poisoning. While irradiation kills most bacteria in meat, pork and poultry, it does nothing to prevent gross fecal and other contamination.

Warnings on the hazards of irradiated food were endorsed in a recent publication, in the world's leading peer-reviewed public health journal, by a wide range of national and international experts including:

Dr. Neal Barnard, President, Physicians Committee for Responsible Medicine, Washington, D.C.

Dr. John Gofman, Emeritus Professor, Molecular and Radiation Biology, University of California, Berkeley, California

Dr. Jay M. Gould, Director, Radiation and Public Health Project, U.S.A.

Dr. Vyvyan Howard, Professor of Pathology, University of Liverpool, U.K.

Dr. David Kriebel, Professor of Epidemiology, University of Massachusetts, Lowell, Massachusetts

Dr. Marvin Legator, Professor of Preventive Medicine, University of Texas, Galveston, Texas

Dr. E. Lichter, Professor of Community Medicine, University of Illinois Medical School, Chicago, Illinois

Dr. William Lijinsky, former Director, Chemical Carcinogenesis, Frederick Cancer Research Center, Maryland

Dr. Sheldon Margen, Emeritus Professor of Public Health Nutrition, University of California, Berkeley, California

Dr. Vicente Navarro, Professor of Health and Public Policy, The Johns Hopkins University, Baltimore, Maryland, Professor of Political and Social Sciences, Universitat Pompeu Fabra, Spain

Dr. Herbert Needleman, Professor of Pediatrics and Psychiatry, University of Pittsburgh, Pittsburgh, Pennsylvania

Dr. Robert Rinehart, Emeritus Professor of Biology, San Diego State University, California

Dr. George Tritsch, Cancer Research Scientist, Roswell Park Memorial Institute, New York State Department of Health, New York

Dr. Quentin Young, past President, American Public Health Association, Chairman, Health and Medicine Policy Research Group, Chicago, Illinois

June 12, 2001

THE AMERICAN CANCER SOCIETY IS THREATENING THE NATIONAL CANCER PROGRAM

Operating behind closed doors and with powerful political connections, Dr. Samuel Epstein, charges the American Cancer Society (ACS) with forging a questionably legal alliance with the federal Centers for Disease Control and Prevention (CDC) in attempts to hijack the National Cancer Program. The ACS is also charged with virtual neglect of cancer prevention.

Dr. Quentin Young, warns: "The ACS political agenda reveals a pattern of self interest, conflicts of interest, lack of accountability and non-transparency to all of which the media have responded with deafening silence".

Among their concerns:

- The National Cancer Act, the cornerstone of the National Cancer Institute's (NCI) war on cancer, is under powerful attack by the ACS, the world's largest non-religious "charity". The plan was hatched in September 1998 when, meeting behind closed doors, the ACS created a "National Dialogue on Cancer" (NDC), co-chaired by former President Bush and Barbara Bush, with representatives from the CDC, the giant cancer drug industry, and Collaborating Partners from survivor advocacy groups. The NDC leadership then unilaterally spun off a National Cancer Legislative Committee, co-chaired by Dr. John Seffrin, CEO of the ACS and Dr. Vincent DeVita, Director of the Yale Cancer Center and former NCI Director, to advise Congress on re-writing the National Cancer Act.
- The relationships between the ACS, NDC and its Legislative Committee raise questions on conflicts of interest. John Durant, former executive president of the American Society for Clinical Oncology, charged: "It has always seemed to me that this was an issue of control by the ACS over the cancer agenda—. They are protecting their own fundraising capacity" from competition by survivor groups. The leading U.S. charity watchdog, The Chronicle of Philanthropy, further concluded, "The ACS is more interested in accumulating wealth than saving lives".
- The ACS-CDC relationship is focused on diverting political emphasis and funds away from NCI's peer-reviewed scientific research to CDC's community programs, which center on community screening, behavioral intervention, and tobacco cessation rather than prevention.

- There are major concerns on interlocking ACS-CDC interests. CDC has improperly funded ACS with a $3 million sole source four-year cooperative agreement. In turn, ACS has made strong efforts to upgrade CDC's role in the National Cancer Program, increase appropriations for CDC's non-peer reviewed programs, and facilitate its access to tobacco litigation money.
- The ACS priority for tobacco cessation programs is inconsistent with its strong ties to the industry. Shandwick International, representing R.J. Reynolds, and Edelman, representing Brown & Williamson Tobacco Company, have been major PR firms for the NDC and its Legislative Committee.
- ACS has made questionably legal contributions to Democratic and Republican Governors' Associations. "We wanted to look like players and be players", ACS explained.
- DeVita, the Legislative Committee co-chair, is also chairman of the Medical Advisory Board of CancerSource.com, a website launched by Jones & Bartlett which publishes the ACS Consumer's Guide to Cancer Drugs; three other members of the Committee also serve on the board. DeVita thus appears to be developing his business interests in a publicly-funded forum.
- The ACS has a longstanding track record of indifference and even hostility to cancer prevention. This is particularly disturbing in view of the escalating incidence of cancer now striking one in two men and one in three women in their lifetimes. Recent examples include issuing a joint statement with the Chlorine Institute justifying the continued global use of persistent organochlorine pesticides, and also supporting the industry in trivializing dietary pesticide residues as avoidable risks of childhood cancer. ACS policies are further exemplified by allocating under 0.1 percent of its $700 million annual budget to environmental and occupational causes of cancer.

These considerations clearly disqualify the ACS from any leadership role in the National Cancer Program. The public should be encouraged to redirect funding away from the ACS to cancer prevention advocacy groups. ACS conduct, particularly its political lobbying and relationship to CDC, should be investigated by Congressional Appropriations and Oversight committees. These committees should also recommend that the National Cancer Program direct the highest priority to cancer prevention.

ENDORSERS:

Quentin D. Young, M.D.
Chairman of the Health and Medicine Policy Research Group
Past President of American Public Health Association
Chicago, Illinois

October 10, 2001

AMERICAN ACADEMY OF PEDIATRICS GUIDELINES FOR TREATING BEHAVIORAL DISORDERS IN CHILDREN WITH RITALIN IGNORES EVIDENCE OF CANCER RISKS

Based on an industry-funded multi-university trial on 282 pre-teen children treated with Ritalin for attention deficit/hyperactivity disorders (ADHD), just published in Pediatrics, the American Academy of Pediatrics has endorsed the use of the drug. However, the Academy ignores clear evidence of the drug's cancer risks of which parents, teachers and school nurses, besides most pediatricians and psychiatrists, still remain uninformed and unaware.

Some 40 years after the drug was first marketed by Ciba Geigy, carcinogenicity tests were conducted at the taxpayers expense by the National Toxicology Program, the results of which were published in 1995. Adult mice were fed Ritalin over a two-year period at dosages close to those prescribed to children. The mice developed a statistically significant incidence of liver abnormalities and tumors, including highly aggressive rare cancers known as hepatoblastomas. These findings are particularly disturbing as the tests were conducted on adult, rather than young mice which would be expected to be much more sensitive to carcinogenic effects. The National Toxicology Program concluded that Ritalin is a "possible human carcinogen," and recommended the need for further research. While still insisting that the drug is safe, the Food and Drug Administration admitted that these findings signal "carcinogenic potential," and required a statement to this effect in the drug's package insert. However, these inserts are not seen by parents or nurses.

The Physicians' Desk Reference admits evidence on the carcinogenicity of Ritalin, now manufactured by Novartis, qualified by the statement that "the significance of these results is unknown," apparently not recognizing that this is more alarming than reassuring. Apart from cancer risks, there is also suggestive evidence that Ritalin induces genetic damage in blood cells of Ritalin-treated children.

Concerns on Ritalin's cancer risk are more acute in view of the millions of children treated annually with the drug and the escalating incidence of childhood cancer, by some 35% over the last few decades, quite apart from delayed risks of cancer in adult life. These risks are compounded by the availability of alternative safe and effective procedures, notably behavior modification and biofeedback.

There is no justification for prescribing Ritalin, even by highly qualified pediatricians and psychiatrists, unless parents have been explicitly informed of the drug's cancer risks. Otherwise, prescribing Ritalin constitutes unarguable medical malpractice.

May 9, 2002

ESCALATING INCIDENCE OF CHILDHOOD CANCER REMAINS IGNORED BY THE NATIONAL CANCER INSTITUTE

Since passage of the 1971 National Cancer Act, the incidence of childhood cancer has steadily escalated to alarming levels. Childhood cancers have increased by 26% overall, while the incidence of particular cancers has increased still more: acute lymphocytic leukemia, 62%; brain cancer, 50%; and bone cancer, 40%. The NCI, besides by the "charitable" American Cancer Society (ACS), have failed to inform the public, let alone Congress and regulatory agencies, of this alarming information. As importantly, they have failed to publicize well-documented scientific information on avoidable causes responsible for the increased incidence of childhood cancer. Examples include:

- Over 20 U.S. and international studies have incriminated paternal and maternal exposures (pre-conception, during conception and post-conception) to a wide range of occupational carcinogens as major causes of childhood cancer.
- There is substantial evidence on the risks of brain cancer and leukemia in children from frequent consumption of nitrite-dyed hot dogs; consumption during pregnancy has been similarly incriminated. Nitrites, added to meat for coloring purposes, have been shown to react with natural chemicals in meat (amines) to form a potent carcinogenic nitrosamine.
- Consumption of non-organic fruits and vegetables, particularly in baby food, contaminated with high concentrations of multiple residues of carcinogenic pesticides, poses major risks of childhood cancer, besides delayed cancers in adult life.
- Numerous studies have shown strong associations between childhood cancers, particularly brain cancer, non-Hodgkin's lymphoma and leukemia, and domestic exposure to pesticides from uses in the home, including pet flea collars, lawn and garden; another major source of exposure is commonplace use in schools.
- Use of lindane, a potent carcinogen in shampoos for treating lice and scabies, infesting about six million children annually, is associated with major risks of brain cancer; lindane is readily absorbed through the skin.

- Treatment of children with Ritalin for "Attention Deficit Disorders" poses risks of cancer, in the absence of informed parental consent. Ritalin has been shown to induce highly aggressive rare liver cancers in rodents at doses comparable to those prescribed to children.
- Maternal exposure to ionizing radiation, especially in late pregnancy, is strongly associated with excess risks of childhood leukemia.

It is of particular significance that the cancer establishment ignored the continuing increase in the incidence of childhood cancer in its heavily promoted, but highly arguable, March 1998 "claim to have reversed an almost 20-year trend of increasing cancer cases."

The failure of the NCI to warn of these avoidable cancer risks reflects mindsets fixated on damage control—screening, diagnosis, and treatment—and basic genetic research, with indifference to primary prevention, as defined by research and public education on avoidable causes of cancer.

The minimal priorities for prevention reflects mindsets and policies and not lack of resources. NCI's annual budget has increased some 20-fold since passage of the 1971 Act, from $220 million to $4.2 billion. NCI expenditures on primary prevention have been estimated as under 4% of its budget.

It should be particularly stressed that fetuses, infants and children are much more vulnerable and sensitive to toxic and carcinogenic exposures than are adults. It should also be recognized that the majority of carcinogens also induce other chronic toxic effects, especially in fetuses, infants and children. These include endocrine disruptive and reproductive, haematological, immunological and genetic, for which there are no available incidence trend data comparable to those for cancer.

The continued silence of the NCI on avoidable causes of childhood, besides a wide range of other, cancers is in flagrant denial of the specific charge of the 1971 National Cancer Act "to disseminate cancer information to the public." As seriously, this silence is a denial of the public's inalienable democratic right-to-know of information directly impacting on their health and lives, and of their right to influence public policy.

ENDORSER:

Quentin D. Young, M.D.
Chairman of Health and Medicine Policy Research Group
Past President of the American Public Health Association

July 11, 2002

PHTHALATES IN COSMETICS ARE SUSPECT, BUT CARCINOGENS EVEN MORE SO

The Environmental Working Group, Coming Clean, and Health Care Without Harm groups are to be warmly commended for their stellar July 10 report on unlabelled phthalate ingredients in common cosmetics and personal care (CPC) products.

In October 2000, the Centers for Disease Control and Prevention and other federal scientists reported on the identification of phthalates in the urine of adults, with highest levels in premenopausal women. The FDA responded that it would "consider" this information. This response was and remains reckless, in view of well-documented evidence since 1985 that phthalates induce birth defects, low sperm counts, and other reproductive toxicity in experimental animals.

A critical 1990 report by the U.S. General Accounting Office, charging that the FDA committed no resources for assessing CPC products safety, had no impact on the agency's reckless policies. The agency's sole requirement is restricted to ingredient labeling of products, except fragrances and perfumes.

However, with rare exceptions such as children's bubble baths, the FDA has never required the industry to label its products with any warning of well—documented risks, particularly reproductive and cancer; nor has the FDA banned the sale of unsafe products to an unsuspecting public, although so explicitly authorized by the 1938 Food, Drug and Cosmetics Act. Examples of carcinogenic products and ingredients include:

Black and dark brown permanent hair dyes contain "coal tar" dye ingredients recognized as carcinogens in experimental animals. This evidence is supported by studies establishing that regular use of these dyes poses major risks of relatively rare cancers-non-Hodgkin's lymphoma, Hodgkin's disease, and multiple myeloma.

Cosmetic grade talc is carcinogenic in experimental animals. Also, frequent genital dusting with talc, routinely practiced by some 17% of premenopausal women, increases risks of ovarian cancer.

A group of widely used preservatives, such as quaternium 15 and bronopol, commonly used in baby products, though not carcinogenic themselves, break down to release formaldehyde, a potent irritant and carcinogen.

Lanolin, widely used on babies' skin and nipples of nursing mothers, is commonly contaminated with DDT and other carcinogenic pesticides. n Commonly used detergents and foaming agents, such as polysorbates and

PEG, are usually contaminated with the volatile carcinogens dioxane and ethylene oxide, although they could readily be removed by vacuum stripping during manufacture.

DEA, another widely used detergent, has been known since 1975 to combine with nitrite preservatives or contaminants in CPC products to form a highly carcinogenic nitrosamine. Furthermore, in 1997, DEA itself was shown to be carcinogenic following application to mouse skin.

Citizen petitions to the FDA by the Cancer Prevention Coalition in 1994 and 1996 detailing evidence on the cancer risks of talc and of DEA-containing products, respectively, and "Seeking Carcinogenic Labeling" on these products, met with no substantive response.

Concerns on cancer risks from CPC products are emphasized by: the unrecognized presence of over 50 carcinogenic ingredients in these products; lifelong use of multiple products by the majority of the U.S. population; the ready skin absorption of many carcinogenic ingredients, further increased by detergents, especially when left on the skin for prolonged periods; and by decades-long suppression of information by FDA and the industry in denial of consumers' democratic right-to-know.

Mainstream industry products thus pose significant public health risks, particularly reproductive and cancer. The role of these avoidable exposures in the escalating incidence of cancer, now striking nearly one in two men and over one in three women in their lifetimes, remains largely unrecognized by our apparently health conscious society. Armed with such information, consumers should protect themselves by shopping for safe alternative products available from the growing non-mainstream industry. Finally, Congress should belatedly and aggressively ensure that the FDA obeys the law.

August 15, 2002

GROUPS CALL FOR LABELING OF COSMETICS AND TOILETRIES, CITING CANCER AND OTHER HEALTH RISKS

Senator Edward Kennedy (D-MA) is to be commended for his May 2002 bill (S. 2499) requiring consumer-friendly food label warnings for allergens, to which roughly 7 percent of the U.S. population are sensitive. Today, a coalition of public health and environmental organizations are requesting Senator Kennedy to consider legislation mandating similar labels for cosmetics and toiletries containing ingredients that pose serious, irreversible health risks.

Millions of Americans are sensitive to allergens in cosmetics, particularly in fragrances and perfumes. However, in addition to allergens, cosmetics and toiletries contain numerous other hazardous ingredients, including almost 100 carcinogens and 15 endocrine (hormonal) disruptors, particularly phthalates.

"These ingredients pose risks of cancer, genetic damage, and reproductive toxicity (including infertility) to unsuspecting consumers, and their infants and children," said University of Illinois School of Public Health Emeritus Professor Samuel Epstein, M.D.

These risks are high. This is due to: the virtual lifelong use of many cosmetic products, such as shampoos and lotions; their routine daily application to large areas of skin; the ready skin absorption of some ingredients, facilitated by detergents in most products; the inhalation absorption of volatile ingredients or their contaminants; and the additive or synergistic interactions between multiple carcinogenic or otherwise toxic ingredients.

Strong concerns on these risks were expressed by Senator Kennedy at hearings on the 1997 FDA cosmetics reform bill. "Our message is that cosmetics can be dangerous to your health.—The American people have a right to full and fair information about the actual and potential dangers of the products they use every day."

Despite these considerations, FDA still denies consumers their right-to-know by refusing to require label warnings on the risks of cosmetic ingredients. This failure violates the 1938 Federal Food, Drug and Cosmetic Act which mandates that "each ingredient used in a cosmetic product—shall be adequately substantiated for safety prior to marketing," and which authorizes FDA to recall and seize unsafe products. Nevertheless, the Agency merely requires a listing of the complex chemical names or their abbreviations of the 10 to 20 ingredients on product labels. However, this information is incomprehensible to consumers, let alone their physicians.

A November 1994 citizen petition to the FDA requested the agency to require that cosmetic talc products be labeled with a warning that frequent application to the genital area significantly increases risks of ovarian cancer. FDA declined to act on this petition on grounds of the "limited availability of resources and other agency priorities."

An October 1996 citizen petition to the FDA requested the agency to require that cosmetics containing the common detergent diethanolamine (DEA) be labeled with a cancer warning, as DEA reacts with nitrites present in many products to form a potent (nitrosamine) carcinogen. DEA itself was also subsequently shown to be carcinogenic when applied to mouse skin. FDA similarly declined to act on this petition.

More seriously, FDA has declined to request Congressional authority to require label warnings on black and dark brown coal tar hair dyes, which are technically exempt from the 1938 Cosmetic Act. This reflects disregard of a series of studies over the last three decades incriminating prolonged use of these dyes with breast and bladder cancers, and non-Hodgkin's lymphoma and multiple myeloma.

FDA policies and those of the Cosmetic, Toiletry and Fragrance Association (CTFA), the U.S. trade association, which represents the multi-billion dollar cosmetic industry, are mutually supportive. The major priority of the CTFA is to prevent "new and unnecessary" label warnings.

Label warnings are even more critical in view of the escalating incidence of cancer, now striking nearly one in two men and more than one in three women in their lifetimes. Still sharper increases are anticipated in coming decades.

Informed by user-friendly labels, consumers could reduce their avoidable risks of cancer and other disease by shunning unsafe products and shopping for safer alternatives. While currently limited, their availability will rapidly increase with increasing demand; this is well exemplified by the organic food industry which has escalated to its current $8 billion market share over the last decade. Legislative action by Senator Kennedy would not only protect consumers, but also stimulate overdue recognition by the $20 billion mainstream petrochemical cosmetic industry that safety sells.

In striking contrast to FDA policies, the Scientific Committee on Cosmetic Products of the European Union recently called for a blanket ban on all carcinogenic, gene-damaging and reproductive toxic ingredients in cosmetics.

Finally, FDA's failure to require the cosmetic industry to disclose information on risks of their products to U.S. consumers is at least as critical as SEC's failure to require disclosure of information on corporate accountability to public investors. Clearly, the FDA is a lap dog, rather than watchdog, of the cosmetic industry.

ENDORSERS:

Mark Helm, Director
Media Relations
Friends of the Earth

Bryony Schwan
National Campaigns Director
Women's Voices for the Earth

Larry Bohlen
Friends of the Earth

Alise Cappel
Center for Environmental Health

Gary Cohen
Environmental Health Fund

Mary Lamielle
National Center for Environmental Health Strategies, Inc.

David Monk
Oregon Toxics Alliance

Barbara Wilkie
Environmental Health Network

Janet Zeller
Blue Ridge Environmental Defense League

November 1, 2002

USDA'S ALLOWING SCHOOLS TO SERVE IRRADIATED MEAT IS RECKLESS

USDA claims that irradiated food is safe, and that low levels of radiation are used do not even pass the laugh test," warned Dr. Epstein. The Parent Teacher Association, nationally, regionally and locally, and parents are urged to boycott irradiated food, and protect children from serious risks to future health and life.

Irradiated meat is a very different product than natural meat. This is hardly surprising as the approved irradiation dosage of 450,000 rads. is some 200 million times greater than a chest X-ray. Apart from high levels of benzene, new chemicals known as "unique radiolytic products" have been identified in irradiated food since the 1970's. Contrary to USDA assurances, which have been rejected by a high level expert FDA committee in addition to independent scientists, these pose risks of cancer, and genetic damage, as demonstrated in test tube, animal tests and also children. Furthermore, as admitted by a USDA report, cooking irradiated food depletes its vitamin content, resulting in "empty calorie food."

Irradiation is now being aggressively promoted by the food industry to divert attention from grossly unsanitary conditions in factory style feedlots, slaughterhouses and packing plants, and to sterilize meat contaminated with feces. The recklessness of the industry is encouraged by recently leaked UDSA instructions which discourage federal meat inspectors from preventing fecal contamination of meat: "Remember YOU are accountable for the very serious responsibility of stopping the company's production for the benefit of food safety."

Our warnings on the dangers of irradiated food are endorsed by some 25 independent national and international experts, and by Public Citizen and other consumer groups.

Sanitation, but not irradiation, is the answer to preventing food poisoning.

May 8, 2003

PUBLIC REMAINS UNINFORMED OF ESCALATING INCIDENCE OF CHILDHOOD CANCER AND ITS AVOIDABLE CAUSES

From 1975 to 2000, the incidence of childhood cancer has escalated to alarming proportions warns the Cancer Prevention Coalition's new report, "The Stop Cancer Before It Starts Campaign." Childhood cancers have increased by 32 percent overall: acute lymphocytic leukemia, 57 percent; brain cancer, 50 percent; kidney cancer, 48 percent; and bone cancer, 29 percent. Childhood cancer is their number one killer, second only to accidents.

The federal National Cancer Institute (NCI) and the American Cancer Society (ACS) have failed to inform the public of the increasing incidence of childhood cancer. Furthermore, the NCI claims that: "The causes of childhood cancers are largely unknown." This is contrary to substantial scientific evidence on their avoidable causes, the wide range of carcinogens to which fetuses, infants, and children are exposed, and their much greater vulnerability than adults. Additionally, most carcinogens cause other toxic effects hormonal or endocrine disruptive, neurological, and immunological.

Avoidable carcinogenic exposures of the fetus, infants, and children fall into three categories:

1. Environmental and Occupational

   - Pesticides: contaminants in drinking water; urban spraying; uses in schools, including wood playground sets treated with chromated copper arsenate
   - Petrochemical and other industrial pollutants: atmospheric emissions; contaminants in drinking water
   - Combustion pollutants: power plants; incinerator stacks; diesel exhaust
   - Radioactive pollutants: atmospheric emissions from nuclear energy plants; contaminants in drinking water
   - Occupational carcinogens: parental exposures during pregnancy

2. Domestic/Household

   - Pesticides: uses in the home, lawn and pet flea collars; contaminants in non-organic food
   - Ingredients and contaminants in lotions and shampoos

- Residence near: hazardous waste sites; chemical and power plants; municipal incinerators

3. Medical

- Radiation: diagnostic X-rays in late pregnancy; high-dose radiation CAT scans of infants and children
- Pediatric prescription drugs: Lindane shampoos; Ritalin, for treatment of attention deficit disorder
- Drugs prescribed during pregnancy: the estrogenic DES; the anti-epileptic Dilantin

NCI's silence on such causes of childhood cancer violates the charge of the 1971 National Cancer Act, launching President Nixon's War Against Cancer, "to disseminate cancer information to the public." This silence is also contrary to NCI's 1998 Congressional testimony that it had developed a public registry of avoidable carcinogens. Not surprisingly, the media remain as uninformed as the public. An April 1, 2003 New York Times article, "Success Stories Abound in Efforts to Prevent and Control Cancer," stated that while amazing progress has been made in treating childhood cancers, "their causes remain a mystery."

Besides the NCI and ACS silence on avoidable causes of childhood cancer, they have failed to provide scientific guidance to regulatory agencies, as reflected in their inconsistent and questionable policies. This is illustrated in the well-intentioned current proposal of the Scientific Advisory Board of the Environmental Protection Agency to develop new guidelines for regulating risks "from Early-Life Exposure to Carcinogens." These proposals, however, are based on attempting to quantify risks from individual carcinogens in air and water, without any recognition of their unpredictable additive or multiplicative effects. These proposals also ignore additional risks from a wide range of other carcinogens, such as those in food and cosmetics, regulated by the Food and Drug Administration, and such, as household products including pesticides, regulated by the Consumer Product Safety Commission. Furthermore, EPA's proposals are flawed by unscientific assumptions, such as that safe levels of exposure to carcinogens can be theoretically quantified, and that risks based on evidence from rodent tests should be downgraded unless their mechanism of action can be shown to be the same as in humans.

The minimal priorities of the NCI and ACS for research and providing the public with information on avoidable causes of childhood cancers reflect imbalanced policies, and not lack of resources. NCI's annual budget has increased some 30-fold, from $220 million to $4.6 billion, since passage of the 1971 National Cancer Act. NCI expenditures on prevention of avoidable causes of cancer have been estimated as under 4 percent of its budget, while ACS has allocated less than 1 percent of its $800 million revenues, apart from $1 billion reserves, to "environmental carcinogenesis."

Clearly, the time for open public debate, and Congressional oversight of national cancer policy is long overdue.

For further details, see the February 2003 "Stop Cancer Before It Starts Campaign" report at www.preventcancer.com; the report has been endorsed by over 100 scientific experts in cancer prevention, and representatives of environmental, consumer, and other activist groups.

May 23, 2003

THE AMERICAN CANCER SOCIETY MISLEADS THE PUBLIC IN THE MAY 26 DISCOVERY HEALTH CHANNEL PROGRAM

In a one-hour special on the "TOP 10 CANCER MYTHS," the American Cancer Society (ACS) claims to set the record straight. However, these claims are seriously flawed.

While admitting that number of people diagnosed with cancer is increasing, the ACS explains this away as due to aging of the population, and the frequency of cancer in the elderly. However, federal statistics adjusted for aging show a 24% increased incidence rate over the last three decades. What's more, most major increases have involved non-smoking related cancers. These cancers include: non-Hodgkin's lymphoma, 87%; thyroid, 71%; testis, 67%; post-menopausal breast, 54%; and brain, 28%. More disturbing is the escalating incidence of childhood cancers: acute lymphocytic leukemia, 62%; brain, 50%; bone, 40%; and kidney, 14%. Of related interest is an analysis of leading causes of death from 1973 to 1999. Cancer has increased by 30%, while mortality from heart disease decreased by 21%.

Worse still, the ACS has failed to inform the public about scientifically well-documented causes of a wide range of non-smoking related cancers. The ACS goes further by dismissing evidence on risks from domestic use of pesticides, although several studies have clearly shown a strong relationship with childhood cancers. In its recommendation for high vegetable, fruit, and grain diets, ACS ignores the fact that these, including baby foods, are highly contaminated with carcinogenic pesticides, while ignoring the availability of safe organic products. The ACS goes even further in dismissing such concerns. In its Cancer Facts and Figures 2002, ACS reassured that cancer risks from dietary pesticides, besides hazardous waste sites, and ionizing radiation from "closely controlled" nuclear plants, are at such low levels as to be "negligible."

The CANCER MYTHS are consistent with its longstanding track record on prevention, policies, and conflicts of interest. In 1978, the ACS refused a Congressional request to support the Clean Air Act. In 1992, the ACS supported the Chlorine Institute by defending the continued use of carcinogenic chlorinated pesticides. In 1993, just before PBS aired the Frontline special, "In Our Children's Food," the ACS came out in support of the pesticide industry. In a damage—control memorandum, sent to some 48 regional divisions and their 3,000 local offices, the ACS trivialized pesticides as a cause of childhood cancer. ACS also reassured the public that food contaminated with carcinogenic pesticides is safe, even for babies.

In 1994, the ACS published a highly flawed study designed to reassure women on the safety of dark permanent hair dyes, and to trivialize the risks of non-Hodgkin's lymphoma, breast, and other cancers as documented in over six prior reports.

Analysis of the 1998 ACS budget revealed that it allocated less than 0.1% of its $700 million revenues to "Environmental Carcinogenesis."

In 2000, it was discovered that the ACS had close ties to PR firms for the tobacco industry—Shandwick International, representing R.J. Reynolds Holdings, and Edelman, representing Brown & Williamson Tobacco Company. These firms were promptly dismissed once the embarrassing news leaked out.

This indifference or hostility of the ACS to cancer prevention is less surprising in view of its pervasive conflicts of interest with the cancer drug, petrochemical, cosmetics, power plants, and other industries.

Not surprisingly, the authoritative U.S. charity watchdog, The Chronicle of Philanthropy, has warned against the transfer of money from the public purse to private hands. "The ACS is more interested in accumulating wealth than in saving lives."

For a detailed critique of the ACS track record and policies, see the Cancer Prevention Coalition February 2003 "Stop Cancer Before It Starts Campaign" report at http://www.preventcancer.com/; the report has been endorsed by some 100 leading experts in cancer prevention, and representatives of consumer, environmental, and activist groups.

February 23, 2004

SPINNING THE LOSING CANCER WAR

In politics, spinning is an art form. Most accept spinning as a fact of life, whether choosing a politician or merely a bar of soap. However, few would accept this gamesmanship for life and death issues of cancer, particularly if the spinning is underwritten by taxpayers.

But, when it comes to the cancer war, the Pollyannaish promises of the federal National Cancer Institute (NCI) and the non-profit American Cancer Society (ACS) are no more reliable than political flack.

Recent headlines in national newspapers, based on NCI and ACS assurances, report that the "Rate of Cancer Deaths Continues to Drop." This reinforces longstanding claims of miracle "breakthrough" treatments, that mortality would be halved by 2000, that the nation had "turned the corner" in the cancer war, and that "considerable progress has been made in reducing the burden of cancer." However, these claims don't even pass the laugh test.

Cancer death rates have remained unchanged since President Nixon declared the 1971 War Against Cancer. Nearly one in two men, and more than one in three women are now struck by cancer. Cancer has become a disease of "mass destruction."

Contrary to the NCI and ACS, the current cancer epidemic is not due to faulty lifestyle—smoking, unhealthy diet, and obesity. American men smoke less today, and lung cancer rates are steadily dropping. In striking contrast, the incidence of environmentally, and non-smoking related cancers has escalated sharply: non-Hodgkin's lymphoma by 71 percent, testes and thyroid cancers by 54 percent each, post-menopausal breast cancer by 37 percent, and myeloid leukemia by 15 percent; various childhood cancers have increased from 20 to 60 percent. For African Americans, the news is worse: incidence rates have increased by up to 120 percent

The escalating incidence of non-smoking adult cancers and childhood cancers is paralleled by the 30-fold increase in NCI's budget from $220 million in 1972 to the current $4.6 billion. The ACS budget has increased from $130 to $800 million, with about $1 billion in reserves. It seems that the more we spend on cancer, the more cancer we get.

The reason we are losing this winnable war is because NCI and ACS priorities remain fixated on damage control—screening, diagnosis, and treatment—and related basic research. All merit substantial funding. However, less funding would be needed if more cancer was prevented, with less to treat.

Responding to criticisms of such imbalanced priorities, NCI now allocates 12 percent of its budget to "prevention and control," and requires its nationwide Centers to have a "prevention component." However, cancer prevention continues to be narrowly defined in terms of faulty lifestyle, and screening, and excludes any reference to avoidable causes of cancer from exposures to industrial carcinogens. These include: contaminants of air, water, food, and the workplace; ingredients in cosmetics and toiletries, and household products, particularly pesticides.

NCI's indifference to such avoidable causes of cancer extends to denial. For example, NCI claims that, "The causes of childhood cancer are largely unknown," in spite of substantial contrary evidence. Similarly, ACS reassures that carcinogenic exposures from dietary pesticides, "toxic wastes in dump sites," and radiation from "closely controlled" nuclear power plants are all "at such low levels that risks are negligible."

Not surprisingly, Congressman John Conyers (D-MI), Ranking Member of the House Judiciary Committee and Dean of the Congressional Black Caucus, recently warned that so much cancer carnage is preventable. "Preventable, that is if the NCI gets off the dime and does its job."

NCI and ACS policies are compounded by conflicts of interest, particularly with the cancer drug industry. In a 1998 Washington Post interview, Dr. Samuel Broder, NCI's former Director, dropped a bombshell: "The NCI has become what amounts to a government pharmaceutical company." Broder resigned from the NCI to become successive Chief Officer of two major cancer drugs companies.

The ACS has a fund raising apparatus which would make any Presidential candidate blush. Apart from public donations, the ACS swims in the largesse of over 300 Excalibur industry donors, each contributing over $100,000 annually. These include over 25 drug and biotech companies, and petrochemical and oil industries. Unbelievably, ACS legislative initiatives are handled by Edelman PR, the major lobbyist of the tobacco industry, and fast food and beverage companies, now targeted by anti-obesity litigation.

Not surprisingly, The Chronicle of Philanthropy, the nation's leading charity watchdog, has charged: "The ACS is more interested in accumulating wealth than saving lives."

The cancer war is certainly winnable, given radical changes in its high command and priorities, and given information on avoidable industrial causes of cancer is provided to the public and Congress. The President has finally conceded the need for an independent commission to investigate misrepresentations that led us into the war on Iraq. We should use a similar commission to investigate the much more lethal failure of the cancer war.

ENDORSER:

Quentin D. Young, M.D.
Chairman of the Health & Medicine Policy Research Group
Past President of the American Public Health Association

July 1, 2004

ENVIRONMENTAL WORKING GROUP REPORT ON PERSONAL CARE PRODUCTS: AMBITIOUS, BUT FLAWED

The Environmental Working Group (EWG) should be commended for its June "Skin Deep" report on personal care products. EWG should also be commended for its FDA petition to recall or issue "warning labels on 356 personal care products" that, as admitted by the industry's Cosmetic Ingredient Review safety panel, "lack sufficient data to support their safe use in personal care products." Regrettably, however, EWG's report is confusing and scientifically flawed.

EWG emphasizes that "only 11 percent of 10,500 personal care products, identified by the industry's trade association, have been publicly assessed for safety." However, this seems an overstatement. Such "suspect" ingredients include: purified water; sodium chloride (table salt); citric acid; natural amino acids; natural botanicals; FDA-approved colorants; and many food additives approved in 1958 by the FDA as "Generally Recognized As Safe."

Moreover, EWG is apparently unaware that substantial information on a wide range of carcinogenic ingredients, carcinogenic contaminants in other ingredients, and ingredients causing dermatitis in most products, marketed by most major companies, has been widely available for nearly a decade. The Safe Shopper's Bible (Macmillan, 1995), which I co-authored, details such information on these unsafe products. The book also provides information on safer products, marketed by smaller companies.

Furthermore, EWG's claim that "consumers and government officials have no way of knowing of ingredients that can be contaminated with impurities linked to cancer" is questionable. This information is admitted, although trivialized, by the Cosmetic Ingredient Review, with particular reference to a large group of detergents (ethoxylates) which, unless purified, are contaminated with potent carcinogenic impurities. More disturbingly, officials of the federal National Cancer Institute are fully aware of such long-standing information, of which they have failed to inform consumers; the American Cancer Society goes still further by virtually dismissing any cancer risks from cosmetics.

EWG's listing of "Carcinogens in Personal Care Products" identifies eight "known and probable human carcinogens." However, no reference is made to talc, identified as a lung carcinogen, following inhalation tests in rodents by the National Toxicology Program in 1993. This is of particular importance in view of the common use of talcum baby powders. Of greater importance are several publications, in leading medical journals since 1982, reporting that frequent use of talc as a genital dusting powder, practiced by about 17% of women, increases risk of ovarian cancer by four-fold.

Based on these concerns, the Cancer Prevention Coalition and the Center for Constitutional Rights filed a 1994 petition to the FDA seeking "Carcinogenic Labeling on all Cosmetic Talc Products." The FDA has remained unresponsive.

EWG's computerized "Skin Deep" report is detailed in two major searchable sections, Find Products You Use, and Customer Shoppers Guide. The Find Products section evaluates 7,500 products sold by many leading cosmetic companies. These products are evaluated on the basis of "Health Concerns," including: cancer; pregnancy problems; safety violations; harmful impurities; penetration enhancers (ingredients which increase skin absorption of other ingredients); unstudied ingredients; and allergies and other health concerns. Products in 25 different categories are each evaluated on the basis of "Top Five Ingredients of Concern."

However, these evaluations are marred by errors of omission and commission:

"Ingredients of Concern," incriminated as posing risks of cancer in different products, include: tocopherol (vitamin E); hydrogen peroxide; acetone; menthol; sodium borate; boric acid; zinc sulfate; propylene glycol; and parabens. However, there is no evidence on the carcinogenicity of these ingredients, although there has been such speculation for parabens.

More puzzling are the Top Five Ingredients incriminated as posing risks of "Allergies and Other Health Problems." These include sodium borate; boric acid; tocopherol; acetone, and silica. However, none of these are known allergens. Also, contrary to EWG, a fragrance is not an ingredient, nor as implied, necessarily allergenic. In fact, fragrances contain mixtures of ingredients, many of which pose no risks of allergy. Moreover, no information is provided as to nature of the unspecified "Health Problems."

Inexplicably, the report omits any reference to ingredients known to induce genetic damage (mutagens), such as aminophenol, hydroquinone, and crotonaldehyde, even though these have been clearly incriminated in recent European Scientific Committee reports.

EWG unfavorably rates all products containing "penetration enhancer" ingredients, which facilitate absorption of other ingredients through the skin. However, this rating extends to most products, as these contain water, and oil or fatty ingredients. These ingredients are necessarily mixed together to form stable solutions, by the addition of detergent (surfactant) ingredients. There are two main types of detergents, sodium or ammonium lauryl sulfate, and a wide range of unrelated ingredients, known as ethoxylates. Most companies avoid the use of sulfate detergents, as they irritate or damage the skin. While purified ethoxylates are not irritants, they are safe "penetration enhancers." However, this is of no concern, unless the product also contains toxic ingredients.

August 6, 2004

HIGH TIME TO LABEL FRAGRANCE ALLERGENS

On July 20, the U.S. House of Representatives passed the "Food Allergen Labeling and Consumer Protection Act of 2003," requiring explicit labeling of eight major allergens in food products. This will make life much safer for about 11 million Americans with food allergies. But why has no such action yet been taken to protect more than twice the number of Americans who develop allergies from unlabeled allergens in fragranced products?

Exposure to these allergens can result in "allergic contact dermatitis" (ACD). This can range from mere itching and transient redness of the skin, to swelling, blistering, and ulceration. ACD is usually localized to the immediate area of the allergen-exposed skin. However, it may spread extensively, and require treatment with antihistamines and cortisone, and even hospitalization; fatal anaphylactic shock has been reported as a rare complication. Inhalation exposure to highly volatile fragrance allergens is also recognized as a cause of asthma in children and adults, particularly those with sensitive airways.

Over 5,000 fragrance ingredients, predominantly synthetic, are commonly used in a wide range of products. These include: household products, such as soaps, cleansers, toilet blocks, sanitary wipes and pads, air fresheners and even pesticides; common toiletries, such as shampoos, aftershave, and cologne, particularly for men, and sunscreens, eye, nail products, hair dyes, and perfumes, particularly for women; and formaldehyde or other preservatives in virtually all fragrances and cosmetics.

Some cosmetics, and other fragranced products, are misleadingly labeled "fragrance-free" if they contain fragrance ingredients, but not the whole fragrance itself. Also, some companies misleadingly label their cosmetics as "hypoallergenic" if they do not contain any of the more common allergens.

However, while the "hypoallergenic" label, and other labels such as "allergy tested" and "safe for sensitive skin," have considerable promotional value, they can mean just whatever any particular company wants them to mean. Manufacturers of these products are not required to do any skin testing to validate such claims, nor to substantiate them to the Food and Drug Administration (FDA). It should, however, be recognized that the Food, Drug and Cosmetic Act authorizes the FDA to declare any product "misbranded" if there is evidence that it contains harmful ingredients.

According to recent U.S. and Danish surveys, the incidence of ACD has increased by about 10 percent over the last decade. This reflects the burgeoning number of cosmetic and fragranced products being marketed, and their increasing use on infants and children, and by men.

Representative Jan Schakowsky, D-Ill., has reintroduced legislation, "The Safe Notification and Information for Fragrances (SNIFF) Act," to amend the Food, Drug, and Cosmetic Act. This requires that allergens in fragranced products be labeled accordingly. More explicitly, the European Parliament has recently proposed that all products containing 26 well-known allergens should be labeled.

In a damage control response to these legislative initiatives, the industry's International Fragrance Association has agreed that information on allergenic ingredients should be made available, but only on request, to dermatologists for diagnostic purposes. However, this "Fragrance On Call List" action continues to deny the public its undeniable right-to-know of major avoidable causes of ACD. Furthermore, the Association has failed to respond to repeated requests for labeling of fragranced products, stating that they contain no known allergens.

Finally, it should be emphasized that allergens represent the tip of the iceberg of a wide range of other unlabeled toxic ingredients in cosmetics and toiletries. While the effects of allergens are almost immediate and obvious, those of carcinogens, gene-damaging and hormonal ingredients can be delayed for decades. As such, they are poorly, if at all, recognizable. Clearly, corrective legislation is well overdue for other toxic ingredients, besides allergens.

October 14, 2004

EUROPE LEADS THE WAY IN COSMETIC PRODUCT SAFETY

At UNESCO Headquarters on Friday, The French Association for Research on Treatments Against Cancer is convening a trans-Atlantic group of leading cancer specialists to present scientific evidence on the role of environmental pollutants as major causes of cancer and other diseases.

Foremost on the agenda is the proposed new chemicals policy for the European Union, known as REACH—Registration, Evaluation and Authorization of Chemicals—an unprecedented complex of regulations for industrial chemicals.

First outlined by the European Commission in 2001, REACH was opposed by the European and U.S. chemical industries, and also by the Bush Administration. A weaker version was offered in 2003, but in view of the drastic rise in deaths from avoidable causes of cancer such as industrial chemicals, the distinguished scientists at this Colloquium will present evidence to show that REACH needs to be strengthened, not weakened.

As the world's largest chemical market, Europe has the ability to act as a catalyst for reform of global legislative policies on the regulation of industrial chemicals. The U.S. government and chemicals industry is closely watching the progress of REACH on its path through the European legislative process. At this critical moment, the experts meeting at UNESCO are engaged in a life and death struggle with cancer and the chemicals that cause this constellation of diseases.

The Colloquium opens with an address by distinguished French oncologist Lucien Israel, MD, who has spent nearly 60 years in the cancer field. He will share the podium with renowned French virologist Dr. Luc Montagnier, best known for his 1983 discovery of the human immunodeficiency virus (HIV), which has been identified as the cause of AIDS.

From the American side of the Atlantic comes Samuel Epstein, M.D., professor emeritus of environmental and occupational medicine at the University of Illinois at Chicago School of Public Health, and a winner of the Right Livelihood Award who chairs the Cancer Prevention Coalition.

Dr. Epstein will give the introductory morning talk on cancer prevention, which will emphasize the escalating incidence of non-smoking related cancers, such as testicular, brain and childhood cancers.

Boston University Professor of Environmental Health Dr. Richard Clapp will offer his perspective on the epidemiological approach to the links between cancer and the environment. Founder of the Massachusetts Cancer

Registry, he now sits on the Governing Council of the International Society for Environmental Epidemiology.

The Colloquium, organized by Dr. Dominique Belpomme of Pesticides Action Network Europe, will hear from representatives of American, Belgian, British, French, and Spanish scientific and citizens' groups such as the Royal Commission on Environmental Pollution, Greenpeace Europe, the WWF, and the European Environmental Bureau, which represents 143 member organizations in 31 countries.

Paul Lannoye of Belgium, a Member of European Parliament representing the Green Group, will address the issues of a Europe facing environmental pollution, and lawyer Corinne LePage of France will advance the idea that polluting is a crime against humanity.

Cancers resulting from occupational exposure, cancer and foods, chemicals in consumer products—a full spectrum of chemical causes of cancer will be considered with the precautionary principle as well as the principle of prevention in mind.

"We have developed a very high dependence on chemicals," European Environment Commissioner Margot Wallstrom told the Second US-EU Chemicals Conference in Charlottesville, Virginia on April 26. "Yet this is not matched by sufficient knowledge about their potential risks and long-term effects, for which we are paying a high price."

"This is not just an issue for European countries," she said. "Chemical safety is a global concern. Countries all over the world are paying a high price for failures to address chemical safety."

Wallstrom has been the point person for the REACH program, which she said is designed to provide the information and safety Europe needs but in a way that is integrated with international efforts. "To facilitate transfer of information, we will be implementing the Globally Harmonised System, which is the UN system for classification and labeling of dangerous substances," she said.

But experts at the Colloquium strongly believe that the current version of REACH is too weak to be effective, and that it has been deliberately weakened at the behest of the chemicals industry on both sides of the Atlantic.

In a detailed 40 page report, "REACH: An Unprecedented European Initiative for Regulating Industrial Chemicals," Dr. Epstein writes, "In striking contrast to EU governments, which have maintained neutral positions, the Bush Administration has encouraged industry to take aggressive opposition to REACH."

Citing articles in the "New York Times," "Environmental Health Perspectives," and other respected publications, Dr. Epstein presents evidence that the Bush Administration is doing its best to undermine the precautionary principle on which REACH is founded, a principle accepted by the European Commission as a "full fledged and general principle of international law."

"Secretary of State Colin Powell, in a March 2002 U.S. "Nonpaper on EU Chemical Policy," warned that the Precautionary Principle would result in "politically motivated bans" of U.S. chemical products, which account for over 20 percent of all U.S. exports.

Dr. John Graham, administrator of the U.S. Office of Information and Regulatory Affairs, and former director of the industry-funded Harvard University Center for Risk Analysis, in a May 18, 2003 speech to EU regulators, stated that the Administration considers the Precautionary Principle "to be a mythical concept, perhaps like a unicorn."

Confidential documents obtained under the U.S. Freedom of Information Act, have revealed that the U.S. State and Commerce Department, the Environmental Protection Agency, and Office of the U.S. Trade Representative, have formed an alliance with Dow Chemical to fight REACH, as reported in the "Wall Street Journal" on September 9, 2003.

"These tactics, however, may backfire," Dr. Epstein writes. "Senator Frank Lautenberg (D-NJ), with other influential Congressional Democrats, is drafting a proposal to overhaul U.S. regulations to resemble the EU's proposed reforms."

The mainstream industry opposition has been mobilized by the American Chemistry Council and the European Chemical Industry Council, each accounting for approximately 30 percent of the world's chemical production. The Trans-Atlantic Business Dialogue has been established to coordinate industry opposition to REACH, Dr. Epstein notes.

A leaked American Chemistry Council memo, made public by the Washington, DC based Environmental Working Group in November 2003, revealed aggressive and well-funded plans to fight laws and regulations based on the precautionary principle.

The Council's public relations campaign is being handled by the firm of Nichols-Dezenhall, which, Dr. Epstein warns, "has hired former FBI and CIA agents to create phony front groups, and spy on environmental activists, including digging through their trash in efforts to smear them."

The industry is fighting against regulation of highly toxic industrial chemicals that REACH would impose.

Under REACH, certain classes of industrial chemicals are regarded as of Very High Concern. They are:

- carcinogens, mutagens, and reprotoxins which are either known or very likely to be toxic to humans

- chemicals that can become widely disseminated in the environment, and which are persistent, bioaccumulative, and toxic, particularly persistent organic pollutants
- chemicals that are very persistent and very bioaccumulative in humans and wildlife for which toxicity data are still unavailable

Many of these chemicals are ingredients or contaminants in pesticides, and in consumer products, including food, cosmetics and household products.

Under REACH, when a company intends to produce or import new and existing chemicals it would be required to prepare a Chemical Safety Report to notify the European Chemicals Bureau, a new body which would be responsible for the classification and labeling of dangerous substances.

The report would include—data on the identity of each chemical; toxicological, and ecotoxicological properties of intended uses; estimated human and environmental exposures; production quantity; proposed classification and labeling; safety data sheet; preliminary risk assessment; and proposed risk management.

This information would be entered into a publicly available database to be managed by the European Chemicals Bureau.

The chemicals notified would be evaluated by testing, and authorization will be granted for a limited number of chemicals of very high concern.

Chemical companies would be required to pay fees for each submission. Overall costs are estimated at: registration: €300 million; testing of 30,000 high production volume chemicals: €2.1B for a total of: €2.4 billion. Administrative costs of approximately €0.4 billion would be recovered on a fee based system.

The first formalized critique of REACH was detailed by the American Chemistry Council in July 10, 2003. "REACH is impractical and too costly," the Council said, and should be replaced by a "risk-based approach." The high costs of REACH would impose a negative impact on innovation and competitiveness of EU industry, the Council warned.

Dr. Epstein says the chemical industry is making exaggerated claims about the costs of REACH, which he says are only 0.05 percent of the chemical industry's €417 billion turnover in 2000. He maintains that these costs are "likely to be dwarfed by costs of poorly recognized public health and environmental impacts to which REACH makes the briefest reference."

The latest REACH proposal "fails to recognize the much higher public health and environmental costs of its drastically weakened regulations," Dr. Epstein warns. He points to "significantly increased . . . incidence of testicular cancer in young men, and allergies over the last decades, for which the underlying reasons have not yet been identified."

The American Chemistry Council objects that REACH is trade restrictive and incompatible with World Trade Organization objectives and international chemical regulations. The Council and its European counterpart say the EU should rely on existing registration and risk management, rather than on REACH.

The opposition to REACH by European and U.S. industry was so strong that the EU was forced to make substantial concessions, which were formalized in its October 2003 legislative proposals. These were jointly developed by Wallstrom and EU Enterprise Commissioner Erkki Liikanen.

Key among these concessions was the reduction of the number of high production volume chemicals for which comprehensive safety testing would be required from 30,000 to 10,000, in spite of what Dr. Epstein calls "minimal available test data on most of them."

Chemicals produced in smaller amounts, from one to 10 metric tons, were exempted from the requirements to produce data on reproductive toxicity and environmental persistence.

But people are getting sick and dying in increasing numbers from exposure to the very chemicals REACH is designed to regulate, chemicals that they are exposed to not just one at a time, but in combination.

This is one of the most serious weaknesses of the latest REACH proposal writes Dr. Epstein. "REACH focuses on the carcinogenic and other toxic effects of individual chemicals," particularly chemicals classified as of Very High Concern, "to the exclusion of well-documented evidence on additive and unpredictable synergistic interactions between individual carcinogens."

Formaldehyde, styrene, and atrazine each is toxic alone, for instance, but when a person is exposed to them at once, their combined toxicity is even greater.

REACH should be strengthened by emphasis that the right-to-know "is an inalienable democratic principle, with the exception of sensitive national security concerns," writes Dr. Epstein. "This right clearly extends to information on avoidable risks of disease and death, and environmental contamination, due to industry practices."

"These rights override claims of trade secrecy and confidentiality," he writes. "It should, however, be recognized that the right-to-know in the EU, besides other nations, is more honored in the breach than the observance. REACH should explicitly acknowledge this right, and detail the mechanism for its widest implementation."

Workers are at greatest risk of high level exposure to industrial chemicals of Very High Concern, and Dr. Epstein is calling on industry to recognize workers' right-to-know information on all such life threatening dangers. Workers must have specific information on the chemical and common name of each carcinogen, and carcinogenic process, he says, and specific information on precautions that can be taken to avoid inhalation and skin exposures.

Among many other recommendations for strengthening the REACH legislation, Dr. Epstein is calling for "independent audits of industry chemical safety dossiers prior to registration under REACH, and independent auditing of industry claims for waiving authorization of chemicals classed as of Very High Concern, based on no "right to concern," or that risks can be "adequately controlled."

"All advisory committees should include representatives of independent expert stakeholders, and meetings should be open to the public," he advises, and "all committee members should fully disclose their conflicts of interest."

He challenges the existing estimated health benefits, of 50 billion over 30 years, saying they do not reflect the escalating incidence of cancer, nor early life exposures due to industrial chemicals.

The environmental benefits should be estimated and recognized, and industry benefits from technological innovation stimulated by REACH also should be estimated and recognized, Dr. Epstein says.

The very existence of the REACH proposal has emphasized the inadequacies of the 1976 U.S. Toxic Substances Act, Dr. Epstein will tell the Colloquium. These U.S. regulations still require testing of only about five percent of chemicals in commerce. "Reflecting such concerns, exacerbated by the deregulation policies of the Bush Administration, progressive Congressional Democrats are now drafting a proposal to overhaul U.S. regulations to conform with those of REACH," he says. These initiatives may extend to state level, and the city of San Francisco is already moving in this direction.

Considering the wide range of exposure of the public to high production volume chemicals, Dr. Epstein is not surprised that many have been identified, particularly in the United States as body burden contaminants in fat and blood of the general population.

These chemicals are in the fat and blood of Europeans too, and European Environment Commissioner Wallstrom is no exception. The results of her personal blood test are now public knowledge and she shared them with participants in the Second US-EU Chemicals Conference.

"Among all the talk of costs, trade barriers, bureaucracy," she said, "the results of the test underline the urgency of cleaning out the chemicals stable."

"A couple of years ago, a British doctor told me that each of us have roughly 300-400 synthetic substances in our bodies, and that these were not present in our grandparents' generation. This got me curious," Wallstrom said.

"Last summer I participated in a limited screening involving three groups of man-made substances brominated flame retardants, PCBs and organo chlorine pesticides," she said. "Of the 77 looked for in this screening, I had 28 in my body, including PCB and DDT, which have been banned in Europe for several decades."

"I was told that my result was below the average of the group tested," Wallstrom said. "The result certainly made me concerned, particularly since I also was told that some of the chemical burden in my body was transferred to my children when I was breast feeding them. And, synthetic chemicals are certainly not something that I want to leave as a legacy with them!"

Reckless industry practices are violations of human rights, and white collar crime. Under REACH, authorization of chemicals of Very High Concern should be denied if safe alternatives are available.

If public support for REACH is forthcoming, when it is introduced to the new European Parliament of 25 member states after the May elections, it will be none too soon for the scientists and nongovernmental organizations at the Paris Colloquium. Cancer is now a leading cause of disease and death in France and the United States, striking nearly one in two men and more than one in three women in their lifetimes.

February 28, 2005

TIME TO PROTECT BABIES FROM DANGEROUS PRODUCTS

From shortly after birth, mothers tenderly wash and pamper their infants with a wide range of baby products. These include soaps, shampoos, lotions, and dusting powders, some of which are used several times daily.

However, how would mothers react if they discovered that these baby products contain a witch's brew of dangerous ingredients? Hopping mad could be a reasonable understatement.

Most disturbing are three groups of widely used ingredients known as "hidden carcinogens"—ingredients which are contaminated by carcinogens, or which break down to release carcinogens, or which are precursors of carcinogens—to which infants are about 100 times more sensitive than adults.

The largest group of hidden carcinogens includes dozens of wetting agents or detergents, particularly PEGs, Laureths, and Cetearenths, all of which are contaminated with the potent and volatile carcinogens ethylene oxide and dioxane. These carcinogens could readily be stripped off during ingredient manufacture, if the industry just made the effort to do so. Another hidden carcinogenic ingredient is lanolin, derived from sheep's wool, most samples of which are contaminated with DDT-like pesticides.

The second group includes another detergent, Triethanolamine (TEA) which, following interaction with nitrite, is a precursor of a highly potent nitrosamine carcinogen.

The third group includes Quaterniums and Diazolidinyl urea preservatives which break down in the product or skin to release the carcinogenic formaldehyde.

Of additional concern is another group of common preservatives, known as Parabens. Numerous studies over the last decade have shown that these are weakly estrogenic. They produce abnormal hormonal effects following application to the skin of infant rodents, particularly male, resulting in decreased testosterone levels, and urogenital abnormalities. Parabens have also been found to accumulate in the breasts of women with breast cancer.

The common use of Talc dusting powder can result in its inhalation, resulting in acute or chronic lung irritation and disease (talcosis), and even death. Additionally, Talc is a suspect cause of lung cancer, based on rodent tests.

Fragrances, containing numerous ingredients, are commonly used in baby products for the mother's benefit. However, over 25 of these ingredients are known to cause allergic dermatitis.

A final ingredient of particular concern is the harshly irritant sodium lauryl sulfate. A single application to adult human skin has been shown to damage its microscopic structure, increasing the penetration of carcinogenic and other toxic ingredients.

Most disturbing is the ready availability of safe alternatives for all these dangerous ingredients (longstanding information on which is detailed on the Cancer Prevention Coalition website, http://www.preventcancer.com). So, why is it that the multibillion-dollar cosmetic and toiletry industry has not acted on this information? The answer is that the major priority of the industry's trade association is "to protect the freedom of the industry to compete in a fair market place." At the same time, the association pursues a highly aggressive agenda against what it claims are "unreasonable or unnecessary labeling or warning requirements." As Senator Edward M. Kennedy (D.MA) stated at 1997 Hearings on the FDA Reform bill: "The cosmetics industry has borrowed a page from the playbook of the tobacco industry by putting profits ahead of public health."

Astoundingly, the interests of industry remain reinforced by the regulatory abdication of the Food and Drug Administration (FDA), in spite of its authority under the 1938 Federal Food, Drug and Cosmetics (FD&C) Act. Clearly, the FDA is the lap dog, rather than the watchdog, of the industry.

Of even greater concern is the reckless failure of the federal National Cancer Institute and the "non-profit" American Cancer Society to inform the public of the avoidable risks of cancer from the use of baby products, especially in view of the escalating incidence of childhood cancers over recent decades. However, the silence of the American Cancer Society is consistent with its over $100,000 annual funding from about a dozen major cosmetic and toiletry industries.

The protracted failure of Congress to enforce FDA's compliance with the FD&C Act has evoked the growing concern of State legislatures. Assemblywoman Judy Chu (D-Monterey Park) of the California Senate Health Committee, recently introduced landmark legislation that requires disclosure of all carcinogenic, hormonal, and otherwise toxic ingredients in cosmetics. Strongly backed by a coalition of consumer, women's, occupational, and church groups, but opposed by powerful mainstream industry interests, the Bill failed to pass. However, this shot over the bows of the reckless mainstream industry marks the beginning of nationwide State initiatives to protect consumers and their babies from undisclosed dangerous products and ingredients. Safe alternative products and ingredients, including organic, are becoming increasingly available from non-mainstream companies.

ENDORSER:

Ronnie Cummins
National Director
Organic Consumers Association

April 10, 2006

NATIONAL SCHOOL LUNCHES: UNSAFE AT ANY EATING

On April 6, a bipartisan Congressional group, with strong support in both Houses, announced plans to introduce legislation amending the National School Lunch Act. This would prohibit the sale in schools of sugary or fatty junk foods, notably soft drinks and French fries.

This initiative officially endorsed longstanding efforts by many school districts to provide only healthy foods, and hopefully reduce the growing incidence of childhood obesity and related diseases.

Enforcement of this initiative would be the responsibility of the U.S. Department of Agriculture (USDA), which is in charge of the current Public School Lunch Program. This extended authority was applauded by the Center for Science in the Public Interest, a national food safety activist group, stating that "The Agency has done a good job with the official school lunch and could do a good job with all other foods." This endorsement may well be warranted nutritionally. However, it certainly is not warranted by the USDA's failure to disclose well-documented scientific evidence on the risks to health of the two school lunch staples, milk and meat.

Much of the nations milk supply comes from cows injected with a genetically engineered variant of their natural growth hormone, technically known as rBGH (recombinant Bovine Growth Hormone). Manufactured by Monsanto, and sold to dairy farmers under the trade name POSILAC. Injection of the hormone forces cows to increase their milk yield by about 10 percent, while making them sick in the process.

Monsanto and the USDA insist that rBGH milk is indistinguishable from natural milk, and that it is safe for children and other consumers. This is scientifically and medically untrue. rBGH milk makes cows sick. Monsanto has been forced to admit to some 20 toxic veterinary effects on its POSILAC label. These include mastitis, resulting in pus cells in milk, and antibiotics used to treat the mastitis. rBGH milk is also chemically, and nutritionally different than natural milk, and is supercharged with excess levels of a natural growth factor (IGF-1), which is readily absorbed through the intestines into the blood. Of major concern is a wealth of longstanding scientific evidence incriminating these excess levels as delayed causes of breast, colon, and prostate cancers.

Reacting to the fully documented scientific evidence on the dangers of rBGH milk, a wide range of nations including all of Europe, Canada, Australia, New Zealand and Japan have banned rBGH milk.

U.S. beef is heavily contaminated with sex hormones. When U.S. beef cattle enter feedlots, sex hormone pellets are implanted under the ear skin, a process that is repeated at the midpoint of their 100-day pre-slaughter fattening period. These hormones increase the weight of the cattle, adding to profits by about $80 per animal.

The hormones in past and current use include the natural estradiol, progesterone, and testosterone, and their more potent synthetic counterparts, zeranol, trenbolone, and melengesterol. The U.S. Food and Drug Administration (FDA) and the USDA have both maintained and still claim that residues of these hormones in meat are safe and within normal limits.

However, confidential industry reports to the FDA, obtained under the Freedom of Information Act, have revealed high residues of the hormones in meat products. Following a single ear implant in steers of Synovex-S, a combination of estradiol and progesterone, their residues in meat were found to be up to 20-fold higher than normal. The amount of estradiol in two hamburgers eaten in one day by an 8-year-old boy could increase his total hormone levels by as much as 10 percent, particularly as young children have very low natural hormone levels.

Increased levels of sex hormones are linked ever more closely to the escalating increase of reproductive cancers in the U.S., 36 percent for post-menopausal breast cancer, 51 percent for testicular cancer, and 88 percent for prostate cancer, since 1975. These concerns have been strongly reinforced by recent evidence, from researchers at Ohio State University, that meat and blood from cattle implanted with zeranol have powerful hormonal effects, which resist cooking.

Europe has viewed longstanding U.S. claims with considerable skepticism. Since 1989, all 25 European nations have banned the sale of beef from hormone-treated cattle.

The national School Lunch Program is a major focus of the current Midwest BioETHICS 2006 (www.bioethics2006.org) conference in Chicago. This culminates in a Tuesday evening session on the critical need for certified organic milk and meat to replace the current dangerous staples. The conference coincides with the national Biotechnology Industry Organization, which aggressively promotes the industrialization of the nation's food supply.

December 16, 2009

RECKLESS INDIFFERENCE OF THE AMERICAN CANCER SOCIETY TO CANCER PREVENTION

Early this month, top Republican Senator Charles E. Grassley sent letters to the American Cancer Society (ACS), besides the American Medical Association (AMA) and 31 other medical advocacy groups, asking them to provide detailed information on tax-deductible funds that they have received from drug and device makers. Such funds have encouraged these organizations to lobby on behalf of a wide range of industries and strongly influence public policy.

Senator Grassley also invited involvement of "whistleblowers interested in establishing communication regarding wrongdoing or misuse of public dollars." However, this wrongdoing still remains unrecognized by policy makers, let alone by the public. As a result, the incidence of a wide range of avoidable cancers has continued to escalate. Meanwhile, well-documented scientific information on their well-documented causes remains undisclosed or ignored by the ACS. (Epstein, S.S. Cancer Gate: How To Win The Losing Cancer War, 2005).

1971   The ACS refused to testify at Congressional hearings requiring FDA to ban the intramuscular injection of diethylstilbestrol, a synthetic estrogenic hormone, to fatten cattle, despite unequivocal evidence of its carcinogenicity, and the cancer risks of eating hormonal meat. Not surprisingly, U.S. meat is banned by other nations worldwide.

1977   The ACS opposed regulating black or dark brown hair dyes, based on paraphenylenediamine in spite of clear evidence of its risks of non-Hodgkins lymphoma, besides other cancers.

1978   Tony Mazzocchi, then senior international union labor representative, protested that "Occupational safety standards have received no support from the ACS." This has resulted in the increasing incidence of a wide range of avoidable cancers.

1978   Cong. Paul Rogers censured ACS for its failure to support the Clean Air Act in order to protect interests of the automobile industry

1982   The ACS adopted restrictive cancer policies, rejecting evidence based on standard rodent tests, which are widely accepted by governmental agencies worldwide and also by the International Agency for Research on Cancer.

1984   The ACS created the industry-funded October National Breast Cancer Awareness Month to falsely assure women that "early (mammography)

detection results in a cure nearly 100 percent of the time." Responding to question, ACS admitted: "Mammography today is a lucrative [and] highly competitive business." Also, the Awareness Month ignores substantial information on avoidable causes of breast cancer.

1992 The ACS supported the Chlorine Institute in defending the continued use of carcinogenic chlorinated pesticides, despite their environmental persistence and carcinogenicity.

1993 Anticipating the Public Broadcast Service (PBS) Frontline special "In Our Children's Food," the ACS trivialized pesticides as a cause of childhood cancer and charged PBS with "junk science." The ACS went further by questioning, "Can we afford the PBS?"

1994 The ACS published a highly flawed study designed to trivialize cancer risks from the use of dark hair dyes.

1998 The ACS allocated $330,000, under 1 percent of its then $680 million budget, to claimed research on environmental cancer.

1999 The ACS trivialized risks of breast, colon and prostate cancers from consumption of rBGH genetically modified milk. Not surprisingly, U.S. milk is banned by other nations worldwide.

2002 The ACS announced its active participation in the "Look Good . . . Feel Better Program," launched in 1989 by the Cosmetic Toiletry and Fragrance Association, to "help women cancer patients restore their appearance and self-image during chemotherapy and radiation treatment." This program was partnered by a wide range of leading cosmetics industries, which failed to disclose information on the carcinogenic, and other toxic ingredients in their products donated to unsuspecting women.

2002 The ACS reassured the nation that carcinogenicity exposures from dietary pesticides, "toxic waste in dump sites, "ionizing radiation from "closely controlled" nuclear power plants, and non-ionizing radiation, are all "at such low levels that cancer risks are negligible." ACS indifference to cancer prevention became embedded in national cancer policy, following the appointment of Dr. Andrew von Eschenbach, ACS Past President-Elect, as director of the National Cancer Institute (NCI).

2005 The ACS indifference to cancer prevention other than smoking, remains unchanged, despite the escalating incidence of cancer, and its $ billion budget.

Some of the more startling realities in the failure to prevent cancers are illustrated by their soaring increases from 1975 to 2005, when the latest NCI epidemiological data are available. These include:

- Malignant melanoma of the skin in adults has increased by 168 percent due to the use of sunscreens in childhood that fail to block long wave ultraviolet light;
- Thyroid cancer has increased by 124 percent due in large part to ionizing radiation;
- Non-Hodgkin's lymphoma has increased 76 percent due mostly to phenoxy herbicides; and phenylenediamine hair dyes;
- Testicular cancer has increased by 49 percent due to pesticides; hormonal ingredients in cosmetics and personal care products; and estrogen residues in meat;
- Childhood leukemia has increased by 55 percent due to ionizing radiation; domestic pesticides; nitrite preservatives in meats, particularly hot dogs; and parental exposures to occupational carcinogens;
- Ovary cancer (mortality) for women over the age of 65 has increased by 47 percent in African American women and 13 percent in Caucasian women due to genital use of talc powder;
- Breast cancer has increased 17 percent due to a wide range of factors. These include: birth control pills; estrogen replacement therapy; toxic hormonal ingredients in cosmetics and personal care products; diagnostic radiation; and routine premenopausal mammography, with a cumulative breast dose exposure of up to about five rads over ten years.

MAJOR CONFLICTS OF INTEREST

Public Relations

- 1998-2000: PR for the ACS was handled by Shandwick International, whose major clients included R.J. Reynolds Tobacco Holdings.
- 2000-2002: PR for the ACS was handled by Edelman Public Relations, whose major clients included Brown & Williamson Tobacco Company, and the Altria Group, the parent company of Philip Morris, Kraft, and fast food and soft drink beverage companies. All these companies were promptly dismissed once this information was revealed by the Cancer Prevention Coalition.

Industry Funding

ACS has received contributions in excess of $100,000 from a wide range of "Excalibur Donors," many of whom continue to manufacture carcinogenic products. These include:

- Petrochemical companies (DuPont; BP; and Pennzoil)
- Industrial waste companies (BFI Waste Systems)
- Junk food companies (Wendy's International; McDonalds's; Unilever/Best Foods; and Coca-Cola)
- Big Pharma (AstraZenceca; Bristol Myers Squibb; GlaxoSmithKline; Merck & Company; and Novartis)
- Biotech companies (Amgen; and Genentech)
- Cosmetic companies (Christian Dior; Avon; Revlon; Elizabeth Arden; and Estee Lauder)
- Auto companies (Nissan; General Motors)

Nevertheless, as reported in the December 8, 2009 New York Times, the ACS responded that it "holds itself to the highest standards of transparency and public accountability, and we look forward to working with Senator Grassley to provide the information he requested."

THE CHRONICLE OF PHILANTHROPY

As the nation's leading charity watch dog, the Chronicle has warned against the transfer of money from the public purse to private hands. It also warned that "The ACS is more interested in accumulating wealth than in saving lives."

A copy of this release has been sent to Senator Charles E. Grassley, of Iowa.

January 26, 2010

PRESIDENT OBAMA AND THE CONGRESS MUST TAKE ACTION ON CANCER PREVENTION

President Obama has pledged to reform the national health care system. Central to this, as the President has stressed, is containing the spiraling costs of health care—costs which are soaring at about six percent each year. Most experts agree that this is not possible without any plan to prevent Americans from getting cancer in the first place. This year, 1.5 million people will be diagnosed with cancer. Of them, 562,000 people, over 1,500 every day, will die.

The cancer epidemic now strikes as many as one in three Americans and takes the life of one in four. After nearly 40 years of losing the war against cancer, a war that President Nixon declared in December 1971, we are taking grossly inadequate action to protect us from this menace.

Based on recent estimates by the National Institutes of Health, the total costs of cancer are $219 billion a year. The annual costs to taxpayers of diagnosis and treatment amount to $89 billion; the annual costs of premature death are conservatively estimated at $112 billion; and the annual costs due to lost productivity are conservatively estimated at $18 billion. And these are the quantifiable, inflationary costs. The human costs surely are of far greater magnitude.

The connection between our losing the cancer war and the need to control ITS costs through prevention is clear. Cancer is not only one of the most costly and sometimes deadly diseases in America, it is also one of the most avoidable.

To be sure, smoking remains the best-known and single largest cause of cancer, particularly lung cancer. While incidence rates of lung cancer in men have declined by 20 percent over the past three decades, rates in women increased by 111 percent. But more importantly, non-smoking cancers—due to known chemical and physical carcinogens—have increased substantially since 1975. Some of the more startling realities in the failure to prevent cancer are illustrated by their soaring rates. These include:

- Malignant melanoma of the skin in adults has increased by 170 percent, mainly due to the use of sunscreens in childhood that fail to block long wave ultraviolet light.
- Thyroid cancer has increased by 116 percent due in large part to ionizing radiation.

- Non-Hodgkin's lymphoma has increased by 80 percent due mostly to phenoxy herbicides, and phenylenediamine black hair dyes.
- Testicular cancer has increased by 60 percent due to pesticides, hormonal ingredients in cosmetics and personal care products; and estrogen residues in meat.
- Childhood leukemia has increased by 55 percent due to ionizing radiation; domestic pesticides; nitrite preservatives in meats, particularly hot dogs; and parental exposures to occupational carcinogens.
- Ovary cancer (mortality) for women over the age of 65 has increased by 47 percent in African American women, and by 13 percent in Caucasian women due to genital use of talc powder.

Breast cancer has increased by 17 percent due to a wide range of causes. These include: birth control pills, estrogen replacement therapy, toxic hormonal ingredients in cosmetics and personal care products, diagnostic radiation and routine premenopausal mammography, with a cumulative breast dose exposure of up to about five rads over 10 years.

It is now beyond scientific dispute that environmental and occupational exposures to carcinogens are the primary cause of non-smoking related cancers. An October 2007 publication on environmental and occupational causes of cancer by one of us (Dr. Richard Clapp) further emphasized that the increasing incidence of cancer is due to preventable exposures to carcinogens in workplace and environment.

This publication summarizes extensive scientific evidence on cancers resulting from environmental exposures to formaldehyde, chlorinated organic pesticides, and organic solvents. It also details evidence attributing the increasing incidence of lung cancers to preventable occupational exposures to a wide range of carcinogens. These include asbestos, formaldehyde, methylene chloride, benzene, and ethylene oxide.

The National Cancer Institute (NCI) is the primary federal agency devoted exclusively to fighting cancer. Paradoxically, the escalating incidence of cancer over the last 30 years parallels its sharply escalating annual budget—from $690 million in 1975 to $6 billion this year. Of this a mere $131 million, 2.2 percent, is allocated to NCI's mission on Prevention and Early Detection. However, in spite of well-documented evidence relating the escalating incidence of cancer to a wide range of avoidable carcinogenic exposures, the NCI remains "asleep at the wheel," and has stubbornly refused to devote significant resources or even attention to prevention.

Major policy changes in the NCI are overdue. These include the appointment of a new Deputy Director for Cancer Prevention, and the allocation of at least 4 percent of the NCI budget to prevention programs for fiscal year 2011.

Furthermore, the NCI has touted the imminent success of new cancer treatments promises that have seldom borne out, and which have been widely questioned by the independent scientific community. For instance, in 2004, Nobelist Leland Hartwell, President of the Fred Hutchinson Cancer Control Center, warned that Congress and the public are paying NCI $4.7 billion a year, most of which is spent on "promoting ineffective drugs" for terminal disease. In fact, the costs of these new biotech drugs has increased over 100-fold over the last decade without any evidence supporting their effectiveness in improving survival rates.

Congress now has an epochal opportunity to reform our health care system and prevent diseases, particularly cancer, from occurring in the first place. By taking some simple steps, Congress should enact prompt and aggressive reforms to prevent cancer.

As members of the independent scientific community, we welcome the Obama Administration's goal of health care reform. But while the Administration has put forward a cancer plan, mistakenly it focuses exclusively on the diagnosis and treatment of cancer, rather than on its prevention. In the past, Congress has also misdirected its attention to cancer relief. The simple truth is that the more cancer is prevented, the less there is to treat. That will also save lives and money.

March 29, 2010

FRANK CONFLICTS OF INTEREST IN THE NATIONAL CANCER INSTITUTE

In March 2010, the White House nominated Nobel Laureate Harold Varmus as Director of the National Cancer Institute (NCI).

As a key advisor to President Obama's 2008 Presidential campaign, Varmus was subsequently appointed Co-Chairman of the President's Council of Advisors on Science and Technology. He was previously President of the New York Memorial Sloan-Kettering Cancer Center.

Varmus has a distinguished track record in basic research on cancer treatment. However, as emphasized by the Cancer Prevention Coalition, this is paralleled by lack of familiarity with mounting scientific evidence on cancer prevention. Two decades ago, he claimed, "You can't do experiments to see what causes cancer—it's not an accessible problem, and not the sort of thing scientists can afford to do—everything you do can't be risky."

In 1995, Varmus, then Director of the National Institutes of Health, struck the "reasonable pricing clause," protecting against exorbitant industry profiteering from the sale of drugs, developed with tax payer money. Varmus also gave senior NCI staff free license to consult with the cancer drug industry.

In this connection, the 2008 edition of Charity Rating Guide & Watchdog Report listed Dr. Varmus with a compensation package of about $2.7 million. This is the highest compensation of over 500 major non-profit organizations ever monitored.

As a past major recipient of NCI funds for basic genetic research, Varmus warned that "reasonable pricing" clauses, protecting against exorbitant industry profiteering from drugs developed with tax-payer dollars, were driving away private industry. So he struck these from agreements between industry and the NCI. As a consequence, Varmus eliminated any price controls on cancer drugs made at the tax-payer expense.

Illustratively, using taxpayers' money, NCI paid for the research and development of Taxol, an anticancer drug, later manufactured by Bristol-Myers Squibb. Following completion of clinical trials, an extremely expensive process in itself, the public paid again for developing the drug's manufacturing process. Once completed, NCI officials gave Bristol-Myers Squibb the exclusive right to sell Taxol at an inflationary price. As investigative journalist, Joel Bleifuss, warned in a 1995 In These Times article, "Bristol-Myers Squibb sells Taxol to the public for $4.87 per milligram, which is more than 20 times what it costs to produce." Taxol has been a blockbuster for Bristol-Myers, posting sales of over $3 billion since its approval in 1992, and accounting for about 40 percent of the company's sales.

Taxol was not the only drug involved in such funding practices. Bristol-Myers Squibb now sells nearly one-third of the approximately thirty-five cancer drugs currently available, often with highly inflated profits, and often developed with taxpayer funds. In 1995, Varmus, a past major recipient of NCI funds for basic genetic research, decided that "reasonable pricing" clauses, protecting against profiteering from drugs developed with taxpayer dollars, were driving away private industry. So he struck these from pricing clauses.

Taxol was not an isolated example. Taxpayers have funded NCI's research and development for over two-thirds of all cancer drugs now on the market. In a surprisingly frank admission, Samuel Broder, NCI Director from 1989 to 1995, stated the obvious: "The NCI has become what amounts to a government pharmaceutical company." Nobel Laureate Leland Hartwell, President of the Fred Hutchinson Cancer Research Center, endorsed Broder's criticism. He further stressed that most resources for cancer research are spent on "promoting ineffective drugs" for terminal disease. In this connection, Memorial Sloan-Kettering's Leonard Saltz estimated that the price for new biotech drugs "has increased 500-fold in the last decade." Furthermore, the U.S. spends five times more than the U.K. on cancer chemotherapy per patient, although survival rates are similar.

As an expert in cancer treatment, Varmus appears unaware that almost 700 carcinogens, to some of which the public is periodically or regularly exposed, have been identified by independent scientists. He also seems to be unaware that the more cancer is prevented the less there is to treat.

On June 15, 2009, a letter to Congressional leaders urging drastic reform of the Obama Cancer Plan to mandate prevention, besides urging the annual publication of a public registry of carcinogens, was released by the five scientists listed below. This letter also listed seven cancers, summarized their avoidable causes, and their increasing incidence since 1975, based on 2005 NCI data:

- Malignant melanoma (mortality) of the skin in adults has increased by 168% due to the use of sunscreens in childhood that fail to block long wave ultraviolet light;
- Thyroid cancer has increased by 124% due in large part to ionizing radiation;
- Non-Hodgkin's lymphoma has increased by 76% due mostly to phenoxy herbicides; and phenylenediamine hair dyes;

- Testicular cancer has increased by 49% due to pesticides; hormonal ingredients in cosmetics and personal care products; and estrogen residues in meat;
- Childhood leukemia has increased by 55% due to ionizing radiation; domestic pesticides; nitrite preservatives in meats, particularly hot dogs; and parental exposures to occupational carcinogens;
- Ovary cancer (mortality) for women over the age of 65 has increased by 47% in African American women and 13% in Caucasian women due to genital use of talc powder;
- Breast cancer has increased by 17% due to a wide range of factors. These include: birth control pills; toxic hormonal ingredients in cosmetics and personal care products; diagnostic radiation; and routine premenopausal mammography, with a cumulative breast dose exposure of up to about five rads over ten years.

However, and as an expert in cancer treatment, Varmus was unlikely to be aware of such scientific evidence, which was not widely recognized until relatively recently.

Based on recent estimates by the National Institutes of Health, the total costs of cancer are about $219 billion each year. The annual costs to taxpayers of diagnosis and treatment amounts to $89 billion; the annual costs of premature death are conservatively estimated at $112 billion; and the annual costs due to loss of productivity are conservatively estimated at $18 billion. The human costs surely are of far greater magnitude. Much of these costs could be saved by cancer prevention.

These concerns regarding Dr. Varmus have been recognized and endorsed by the following leading national experts on cancer prevention:

Rosalie Bertell, Ph.D.
Regent, International Physicians for Humanitarian Medicine

Janette D. Sherman, MD
New York Academy of Science, 2009

Quentin D. Young, MD
Chairman, Health and Medicine Policy Research Group

May 4, 2010

CANCER PREVENTION COALITION URGED SUPPORT OF THE SAFE CHEMICALS ACT

The Cancer Prevention Coalition encouraged people to support the Safe Chemicals Act of 2010, introduced by Senator Frank Lautenberg (D-NJ) on April 15 this year. This amends the 1976 Toxic Substances Control Act by requiring manufacturers to prove the safety of chemicals before they are marketed. Of particular concern are carcinogens, to which the public had been dangerously exposed and uninformed for nearly four decades. President Richard Nixon declared the national "war against cancer," and the National Cancer Act was passed. This charged the National Cancer Institute (NCI) "to disseminate cancer information to the public."

The 1971 Act also authorized the President to appoint the director of NCI and control its budget, thus bypassing the scientific and budgetary authority of the director of 26 other National Institutes of Health (NIH).

As a result of this anomaly, NCI's current $5.3 billion budget, 17% that of the entire NIH, remains beyond control of NIH's director. However, the NCI's special status of the NCI was challenged in 2003 by the National Academy of Sciences, at hearings of the House Energy and Commerce, and also by the Senate Health, Education, Labor and Pensions Committees.

Furthermore, contrary to the specific requirements of the 1971 Act, the NCI has still failed to "disseminate cancer information to the public," and to warn the public of a wide range of avoidable causes of cancer.

The 1988 amendments to the National Cancer Program called for "an expanded and identified research program for the prevention of cancer caused by occupational or environmental exposure to carcinogens." However, these amendments have been and remain ignored by the NCI.

For over four decades, NCI policies have been and remain fixated on damage control—screening, diagnosis, treatment and related research. Meanwhile priorities for prevention, from avoidable exposures to carcinogens in air, water, consumer products, and the workplace have remained minimal.

To be sure, smoking remains the best-known and single largest cause of cancer, particularly lung cancer. However, while lung cancer incidence rates in men have declined by 20% over the past three decades, those in women have increased by 111%. But more importantly, non-smoking cancers—due to known chemical and physical carcinogens—have increased substantially since 1975.

Some of the more startling realities in the failure to prevent cancer are illustrated by their soaring increases. Examples include:

- Childhood leukemia has increased by 55% due to ionizing radiation; domestic pesticides; nitrite preservatives in meats, particularly hot dogs; and parental exposures to occupational carcinogens;
- Malignant melanoma of the skin in adults has increased by 168% due to the use of sunscreens in childhood that fail to block long wave ultraviolet light;
- Thyroid cancer has increased by 124% due in large part to ionizing radiation;
- Non-Hodgkin's lymphoma has increased 76% due mostly to phenoxy herbicides; and phenylenediamine hair dyes;
- Testicular cancer has increased by 49% due to pesticides; hormonal ingredients in cosmetics and personal care products; and estrogen residues in meat;
- Ovary cancer (mortality) for women over the age of 65 has increased by 47% in African American women and 13% in Caucasian women due to genital use of talc powder;
- Breast cancer has increased 17% due to a wide range of factors. These include: birth control pills; estrogen replacement therapy; toxic hormonal ingredients in cosmetics and personal care products; diagnostic radiation; and routine premenopausal mammography, with a cumulative breast dose exposure of up to about five rads over ten years. Reflecting these concerns, Representatives Debbie Wasserman-Schultz and Henry Waxman have introduced bills promoting educational campaigns, including teaching regular breast self examination to high school students.

Paradoxically the escalating incidence of cancer over the last thirty years parallels its sharply escalating annual budget, from $690 million in 1975 to $5.2 billion this year. Of this, a mere $314 million (6%) is claimed to be allocated to NCI's mission on "Cancer Prevention and Control."

However, in spite of well-documented evidence relating the escalating incidence of cancer to a wide range of avoidable carcinogenic exposures, the NCI remains "asleep at the wheel," and has recklessly refused to devote significant resources to prevention.

The NCI has also ignored proddings from Congress and independent scientific experts to develop a comprehensive registry of carcinogens. Worse still, the NCI has misled the public by claiming that most cancers are due to 'unhealthy behavior,' blaming the victim, despite overwhelming evidence to the contrary.

For instance, the NCI still claimed that 94% of all cancers are due to "unhealthy behavior," such as smoking, poor nutrition, inactivity, obesity and over exposure to sunlight, while a mere 6% are attributable to environmental and occupational exposures.

These estimates are based on those published in 1981 by the late U.K. epidemiologist Richard Doll. However, from 1976 to 1999, Doll had been a closet consultant to U.K. and U.S. industries, including General Motors, Monsanto and the asbestos industry. Following revelation of these conflicts of interest, just prior to his death in 2002, Doll admitted that most cancers, other than those related to smoking and hormones, "are induced by exposure to chemicals often environmental."

Furthermore the NCI has touted the imminent success of new cancer treatments, but says these promises have seldom borne out, and have been widely questioned by the independent scientific community.

For instance, Nobel Laureate Leland Hartwell, President of the Fred Hutchinson Cancer Control Center, warned in 2004 that Congress and the public are paying NCI $4.7 billion a year, most of which is spent on "promoting ineffective drugs" for terminal disease.

Based on recent estimates by the National Institutes of Health, the total costs of cancer have now reached $228 billion a year. The annual costs to taxpayers of diagnosis and treatment amount to $93 billion; the annual costs of premature death are conservatively estimated at $116 billion; and the annual costs due to lost productivity are conservatively estimated at $19 billion. These are quantifiable and inflationary economic costs. The human costs surely are of far greater magnitude.

May 7, 2010

PROTECT CHILDREN'S HEALTH FROM BISPHENOL-A

On May 7, 2010, I urged public support for the Toxic Chemicals Safety Act of 2010, which established a program to review and protect children from risks of toxic exposures, including Bisphenol-A (BPA), a common contaminant in consumer goods.

On March 30 that year, the Washington Post announced that the Environmental Protection Agency listed BPA as "a chemical of concern." The Post also noted that the U.S. Food and Drug Administration (FDA) previously expressed "concerns about the chemical's hormonal effect on human health." However, the American Chemistry Council claims "that BPA is not a risk to the environment at current low levels."

BPA is widely used in polycarbonate bottles, such as baby products, besides adult personal care and cosmetic products, food can linings, microwave oven dishes, dental sealants, and also medical devices. There are also other major sources of BPA such as cash register and credit-card receipts, which are coated with microscopic powdered BPA, and which many of us handle daily.

A 2007 review of about 700 studies on BPA, published in the journal Reproductive Toxicology, found that the fetus and infants are highly vulnerable to the toxic hormonal effects of this ingredient, technically known as "endocrine disruptive."

Dr. Epstein cites an accompanying study by National Institutes of Health researchers in the same journal, reported uterine damage in newborn rodents exposed to levels of BPA comparable with those of normal human exposure. "This finding may also implicate BPA as a cause of reproductive tract disorders in women, after their earlier exposure as fetuses or infants," he warns.

Previous studies in the journal Endocrinology, and elsewhere, reported that BPA masculinizes the brain of female mice and feminizes the brain of male mice. Toxic effects of this hormone disrupter in pregnant women are evidenced in their infant baby boys by the reduction in the normal distance between their anus and genitals. This decrease in anogenital distance is also associated with a decrease in sperm production.

Based on such evidence, Health Canada declared BPA to be a "toxic chemical" in early 2008.

In addition to these toxic effects, exposure of pregnant rodents to BPA, at levels 2,000 times lower than the Environmental Protection Agency's "safe dose," resulted in sexual abnormalities in their offspring. Dr. Epstein warns that these abnormalities include an increased number of "terminal end buds" in breast tissue, which are associated with a subsequent high risk of breast cancer. However, an American Plastics Council spokesman claimed that the human relevance of these findings is only "hypothetical."

Dr. Epstein warns that BPA has also been found in human blood, placental and fetal tissue, and incriminated as a predisposing factor for prostate cancer. "The authors of this study also linked endocrine-dependent human cancers, such as breast cancer, to the minimal levels of BPA to which pregnant women are exposed," he says.

An August 2, 2007 consensus statement by several dozen scientists warned that BPA, even at very low exposure levels, is probably responsible for many human reproductive disorders.

A September 2008 publication, Endocrine-Related Cancer, by Dr. Gail Prins reviewed the substantial scientific evidence on the toxic hormonal effects of BPA, besides other endocrine disruptive chemicals (EDCs) in pregnant women. She concluded that children are highly sensitive to their toxic effects, particularly subsequent risks of prostate cancer.

In October 2008, Science Daily reported on an article on BPA called "A Plastic World," in a then pending special section on Environmental Research. Two other articles reported that fetal exposure to BPA disrupted the normal development of the brain and behavior in rats and mice. Other articles have also reported that BPA is massively contaminating the oceans and harming aquatic wildlife.

The June 2009 Endocrine Disruption Act authorized the National Institute of Environmental Health Science "to coordinate" research on hormone disruption to prevent exposure to chemicals "that can undermine the development of children before they are born and cause lifelong impairment of their health and function."

This bill was supported by public health, consumer and children's advocacy groups, and further strengthened by California's Senator Dianne Feinstein's legislation to ban BPA from food and beverage containers. Of major relevance, this legislation has also been endorsed by the April 2010 President's Cancer Panel On "Reducing Environmental Cancer Risk: What We Can Do Now," 2008-2009 Annual Report. This report further warns that "to a disturbing extent, babies are born pre-polluted."

There are safe alternatives to BPA. As emphasized in the Dr. Sam Epstein's 2009 book Toxic Beauty, the recent development of "green chemistry" has encouraged the phase-out of product packaging that relies on petrochemical plastic containers, particularly those containing BPA. These containers are now being replaced with biodegradable substitutes, including recycled paper. Such "green" packaging reduces energy use, greenhouse gases, and non-degradable or poorly degradable wastes currently disposed of in landfills.

In January this year, the FDA announced an "Update on BPA," with particular reference to its use in food packaging, plastic baby bottles, feeding cups, and metal containers, to avoid childhood exposure. However, FDA has still not taken any regulatory action to this effect. Meanwhile, Dr. Epstein says, the industry's Cosmetic Ingredient Review Panel does not even make any reference to BPA in its annual "safety assessments."

On April 15, Congressmen Bobby Rush and Henry Waxman released a draft of the Toxic Chemicals Safety Act of 2010. The key provisions of this Act include establishment of a program to review and protect children from risks of toxic exposures, including BPA.

Dr. Epstein says, "The passage of this legislation is urgently needed in order to ban BPA from food packaging and other consumer products, especially to prevent any further childhood exposure."

January 4, 2011

UNRECOGNIZED DANGERS OF FORMALDEHYDE

A December 10, 2010 a two page article in *The New York Times*, "When Wrinkle-Free Clothing Also Means Formaldehyde Fumes," stated that "formaldehyde is commonly found in a broad range of consumer products." These include sheets, pillow cases and drapes, besides "personal care products like shampoos, lotions and eye shadows." It was stated in this article that "most of the 180 items tested, largely clothes and bed linens, had low or undetectable levels of formaldehyde that met voluntary industry guidelines." Most consumers will probably never have a problem with exposure to formaldehyde," since such low levels "are not likely to irritate most people," other than those wearing wrinkle-resistant clothing. "The U.S. does not regulate formaldehyde levels in clothing. Nor does any government agency require manufacturers to disclose the use of this chemical on labels."

On March 5, 2008, Senators Bob Casey, Sherrod Brown and Mary Landrieu introduced an amendment to the Consumer Product Safety Commission (CPSC) reform bill "that would help protect Americans from dangerous levels of formaldehyde in textiles including clothing." The Senators referred to a 1997 CPSC report on formaldehyde, which admitted that "it causes cancer in tests on laboratory animals, and may cause cancer in humans." Accordingly, the senators requested the CPSC to "regulate and test formaldehyde in textiles and protect consumers from this poison."

In August 2010, a Government Accountability Office (GAO) report warned that "a small proportion of the U.S. population does have allergic reactions to formaldehyde resins on their clothes." However, the GAO made no recommendations for any regulatory action.

It is surprising that many people are unaware of the longstanding scientific evidence on the carcinogenicity of formaldehyde. However, this had been detailed in five National Toxicology Program Reports on Carcinogens from 1981 to 2004. These classified formaldehyde as "reasonably anticipated to be a human carcinogen," based on limited evidence of carcinogenicity in humans, and sufficient evidence in experimental animals. This evidence was confirmed in a series of reports by the prestigious International Agency for Research on Cancer (IARC). Its 2006 and 2010 reports explicitly warn that formaldehyde is "a known cause of leukemia in experimental animals—and nasal cancer" in humans.

"Strong" evidence of the nasal cancer risk was also cited in the May 2010 President's Cancer Panel report, "Environmental Cancer Risk: What Can We Do Now?" Nevertheless, and in spite of this explicit evidence, a September

2010 Government Accountability Office report attempted to trivialize the cancer risks of formaldehyde on the alleged grounds that exposure levels are low or "non-detectable."

Of further concern, occupational exposure to formaldehyde has been associated with breast cancer deaths in a 1995 National Cancer Institute report, while environmental exposure has been associated with an increased incidence of breast cancer in a 2005 University of Texas report.

None of the dermatologists quoted in *The New York Times* appear aware of longstanding evidence that most cosmetics and personal care products, commonly used daily by most women, besides on their infants and children, and to a lesser extent men, contain up to eight ingredients which are precursors of formaldehyde. These include diazolidinyl urea, metheneamine and quaterniums, each of which readily breaks down on the skin to release formaldehyde. This is then readily absorbed through the skin, and poses unknowing risks of cancer to the majority of the U.S. population.

January 24, 2011

DANGER OF BONE CANCER FROM FLUORIDE IN TOOTHPASTE, AND DRINKING WATER

As reported in the January 13, 2011 New York Times, Senator James Inhofe (R-OK) warned the U.S. Environmental Protection Agency (EPA) that the move to phase out a fluoride-based pesticide "could create unintended consequences for public health, food safety, and the economy."

Cancer Prevention Coalition Chairman Samuel S. Epstein, M.D. said today that Senator Inhofe may be right about such possible "unintended consequences."

"However," said Dr. Epstein, "he is unaware that these consequences would be clearly beneficial, as they protect against the risks of bone cancer from the use of fluoride in most brands of toothpaste to prevent cavities, and from the fluoridation of drinking water."

In 1977, the National Academy of Sciences expressed concerns on the strong relation between the fluoridation of drinking water and risks of bone cancer to young boys, Dr. Epstein points out.

A decade later, the International Agency for Research on Cancer reported that fluorides in drinking water induced bone cancer in rats. This finding was confirmed by the National Toxicology Program in its 1989, 1990, and 1991 reports.

"Not surprisingly, Procter & Gamble, the leading manufacturer of fluoridated toothpastes, denied that these results were statistically significant," Dr. Epstein said today. "Surprisingly, the Food and Drug Administration (FDA) supported this claim."

Well-documented evidence links bone cancer to fluoride exposure, Dr. Epstein advises.

In 1990, the National Cancer Institute (NCI) reported that, based on an analysis of 1973 to 1987 data, the incidence of a bone cancer, known as osteosarcoma, was increased in males under the age of 20 living in areas where the drinking water was fluoridated. Not surprisingly, this was promptly denied by Procter & Gamble, the major manufacturer of fluoridated toothpaste.

In 1992, the New Jersey Department of Health published a study confirming higher rates of bone cancer in young boys living in fluoridated versus non-fluoridated areas of the state.

A 1993 independent analysis of the 1990 NCI data confirmed excess risks and deaths from bone cancer in young boys exposed to fluoride. These findings were confirmed in a 2001 report by the Harvard School of Dental

Medicine. In 2006, a Harvard University team of scientists published a study reporting a five-fold increased risk of bone cancer in teenage boys who had drunk fluoridated water between the ages of 6 and 8. Apart from exposure to fluoride in drinking water, these finding also incriminated fluoride commonly added to toothpaste.

In July 1997, the Washington Post published an article "Toothpaste: How Safe." This noted that the label of Crest toothpaste carried a small print warning: "If you accidentally swallow more than used for brushing, seek professional help or contact a poison control center immediately." Warning labels to this effect had also been required by the FDA in April that year. The Post article further warned that children age 4 to 6 usually swallow some toothpaste when brushing, rather than spitting it out and rinsing.

"Concerns on fluoride as a major avoidable cause of bone cancer are further and urgently validated by its unrecognized 20 percent increased incidence in children under the age of 15 over the last three decades," Dr. Epstein warns, "as documented in the 1975-2007 National Cancer Institute Surveillance Epidemiology and End Results (SEER) report."

As currently emphasized by Chris Neurath, research director of the American Environmental Health Studies Project, these concerns are all the more critical as 200 million citizens of all ages are still drinking fluoridated water.

Apart from bone cancer, and as warned by the Fluoride Action Network (FAN) last week, "24 studies have shown an association between exposure to moderate to high levels of fluoride in drinking water and lower IQ (and brain damage) in children."

Dr. Epstein says, "A ban by the FDA on fluoridated toothpaste is well overdue, as is a ban by the EPA on the fluoridation of drinking water."

November 18, 2011

THE AMERICAN CANCER SOCIETY IGNORES EVIDENCE ON AVOIDABLE CAUSES OF CHILDHOOD CANCERS

The American Cancer Society (ACS) 2011 annual report "Cancer Facts & Figures" ignores well-documented scientific evidence on the industrial and environmental causes of childhood and wide range of other cancers.

The report lists 13 "Selected (Adult) Cancers," and summarized their known "risk factors," or causes. Overwhelmingly, these were attributed to longevity, obesity, alcohol, smoking, and family history. However, the ACS made no reference to the wide range of avoidable exposures to industrial carcinogens in air, water, food, and the workplace.

The ACS also ignored well-documented scientific evidence on the known industrial and environmental causes of the very wide range of cancers. However, such evidence has been fully documented since 1972, in about 100 reports on individual and groups of carcinogens, by the International Agency for Research on Cancer.

Furthermore, the 2008-2009 Annual Report of the President's Cancer Panel, released in April 2010, included a "Summary of Environmental and Occupational Links with Cancer." This report documented "strong" evidence on cancer risks from exposures to 15 individual or groups of carcinogens, such as talc powder, ethylene oxide, and dioxane. The report also documented "suspected" evidence from exposure to about 40 other individual or groups of carcinogens.

Worse still, that threat of cancer begins even before a birth, and extends beyond dental radiation. Once a pregnant woman absorbs ingredients from the cosmetics and personal care products that she uses, they penetrate through her skin to varying degrees. They then reach the fetus through the approximately 300 quarts of blood pumped daily between the placenta and fetus. Studies on umbilical and blood cord samples have also identified other ingredients, such as triclosan, which are commonly added to deodorants, toothpaste, and cosmetics.

Not surprisingly, the overall incidence of childhood cancers has increased by about 40 percent over the past three decades. Could it have anything to do with the cancer causing (carcinogenic) ingredients in personal care products targeting infants and children which have crowded supermarket and other store shelves over the same period?

In fact, babies are about 100 times more sensitive to carcinogens than are adults. Infants and young children have immature liver enzymes, which give them only limited ability to detoxify the carcinogens besides other toxic ingredients in products which are applied to their skin.

Added to that is the fact that the ingredients in the products that mothers apply to the skin of their infants and children are readily absorbed into their blood and bodies. So, there is every reason why we should be highly cautious about the products that we buy for our infants and children, let alone ourselves.

Also, as infants' and children's cells divide much more rapidly than those of adults, they are much more sensitive to carcinogens, and much more vulnerable to developing cancer later in their lives. No wonder that the overall incidence of childhood cancers since 1975 has increased by 34%, while the incidence of kidney cancer and acute lymphocytic leukemia has increased by about 60%.

Most of us would like to believe that any products, especially those marketed for infants and children, must be safe as otherwise they would never be sold. Surely, the U.S. Food and Drug Administration, the responsible agency of government, let alone the industry concerned, must be looking out for the health of our most vulnerable citizens. Right? No, wrong.

December 15, 2011

MULTIPLE CARCINOGENS IN JOHNSON & JOHNSON'S BABY SHAMPOO

The Cancer Prevention Coalition today congratulated the Campaign for Safe Cosmetics for securing a 11/15/11 agreement with Johnson & Johnson "for reducing or gradually phasing out—trace amounts of potentially cancer-causing chemicals" from Baby Shampoo, "one of its signature products." However, this agreement is limited and restricted to the U.S. market.

There are two carcinogenic ingredients in Johnson & Johnson's Baby Shampoo, dioxane and quaternium 15.

Dioxane is a well-recognized contaminant in alcohol ethoxylates, a group of four ingredients, laureths, oleths, polyethylene glycol and polysorbates. Quaternium-15 is a precursor of two carcinogens, formaldehyde and nitrosamine. Johnson & Johnson has committed to "reducing or gradual phasing out" dioxane and quaternium-15 in their U.S., but not in their international, products.

However limited, Johnson & Johnson's response is in sharp and disturbing contrast to the silence of the Food and Drug Administration (FDA).

This federal agency has still failed to enforce the explicit requirements of the 1938 Federal Food Drug and Cosmetic Act, Dr. Epstein points out. This directs the FDA to require that "the label of a cosmetic product shall bear a warning statement to prevent a health hazard that may be associated with the product."

The regulatory failure of the FDA extends to its failure to respond to the Cancer Prevention Coalition's extensively documented 1996 Citizen Petition "Seeking A Cancer Warning On Cosmetic Products Containing (the carcinogen) Diethanolamine."

Tthe FDA's regulatory failure extends still further to the Coalition's 2008 Petition, "Seeking A (ovarian) Cancer Warning On Talc Products Used By Premenopausal for Women's Genital Dusting."

Both Petitions, endorsed by leading cancer prevention experts, requested the FDA to ban or suspend approval of these products which still pose an "Imminent Hazard," or minimally to require their labeling with a "Caution" or other such warning. However, the FDA has still failed to respond.

Concerns on the cancer risks of talc, dioxane, formaldehyde, nitrosamine, and ethylene oxide, besides other prohibited and restricted carcinogenic ingredients in cosmetics and personal care products, are not new. They were detailed in my 2001 "Unreasonable Risk: How To Avoid Cancer From Cosmetics and Personal Care Products," and 2009 "Healthy Beauty" books.

As published in the February 25, 2011 Science Insider editorial, "Advancing Regulatory Science," FDA Commissioner, Dr. Margaret Hamburg, claimed that FDA's regulations must be based on "better predictive models—functional genomics, proteomics, and metabolomics," rather than "high dose animal [carcinogenicity] studies—unchanged for decades."

Dr. Hamburg's dismissal of standard carcinogenicity tests is bizarre. Their scientific validity has been endorsed by other Federal regulatory agencies, the National Toxicology Program, the International Agency for Research on Cancer, besides the April 2010 President's Cancer Panel.

Furthermore, as stipulated in the 1938 Federal Food Drug and Cosmetic Act, the FDA is charged with regulating food, drugs, and cosmetics based on standard toxicology and carcinogenicity tests. Moreover, the FDA is not charged with, let alone capable of developing irrelevant 'tests that incorporate the mechanistic underpinnings of disease.

As warned by Senator Edward Kennedy at the 1997 Senate Hearings on the FDA Reform Bill, "The cosmetics industry has borrowed a page from the playbook of the tobacco industry by putting profits ahead of public health."

This warning remains current.

APPENDIX A:

THE STOP CANCER BEFORE IT STARTS CAMPAIGN: HOW TO WIN THE LOSING WAR AGAINST CANCER

SPONSORS AND ENDORSERS

February 2003

SPONSORS

Nicholas Ashford, Ph.D., J.D.,
Professor, Technology and Policy, Massachusetts Institute of Technology, Member, Governing Board (Massachusetts) Alliance for a Healthy Tomorrow, and CPC Board of Directors
nashford@mit.edu

Kenny Ausubel,
President, Bioneers, and the Collective Heritage Institute
kenny@bioneers.org

Barry Castleman, Ph.D.,
Environmental Consultant, and
CPC Board of Directors
bcastleman@earthlink.net

Edward Goldsmith, M.A.,
Publisher, The Ecologist, and CPC Board of Directors
teddy.goldsmith@virgin.net

JeffreyHollender,
President, Seventh Generation
jeffrey@seventhgeneration.com

Anthony Mazzocchi
Founder of The Labor Party, and Member
of the Debs-Jones-Douglass Labor Institute, and CPC Board of Directors

Horst M. Rechelbacher,
Founder, Aveda
Corporation, and President, Intelligent Nutrients
horst@intelligentnutrients.com

Quentin Young, M.D., Chairman, Health and Medicine Policy Research Group, National Coordinator of the Physicians for a National Health Program
Past President of the American Public Health Association, and CPC Board of Directors
quentin@pnhp.org

ENDORSEMENTS

Winfield J. Abbe, Ph.D.
Former Associate Professor Physics, University of Georgia
Cancer prevention activist, Athens, GA
wjabbe@aol.com

Thomas J. Barnard, M.D., CCFP, FAAFP
Adjunct Professor of Family Medicine, University of Western Ontario, Canada
Adjunct Professor of Human Biology and Nutritional Sciences, University of Guelph, Ontario, Canada
barnard@mnsi.net

Maude Barlow
National Chairperson, The Council of Canadians, Ottawa, Ontario, Canada
Director, International Forum on Globalization
mbarlow8965@rogers.com

Gregor Barnum
Executive Director, The Household Toxins Institute, Burlington, VT
gregor@seventhgeneration.com

Rosalie Bertell, Ph.D.
President, International Institute of Concern for Public Health, Toronto, Canada
rosaliebertell@greynun.org

Brent Blackwelder, Ph.D.
President, Friends of the Earth, Washington, D.C.
bblackwelder@foe.org

Judy Brady
GreenAction, and Toxic Links Coalition, San Francisco, CA
Member, CPC Board of Directors
jibasmil@aol.com

Elaine Broadhead
Environmental Activist, Middlesburg, VA
elainebroadhead@yahoo.com

James Brophy
Occupational Health Clinics for Ontario Workers, Ontario, Canada
jimbrophy@yahoo.com

Chris Busby, Ph.D., MRSC
Scientific Secretary, European Committee on Radiation Risks
Member, U.K. Government Committee on Radiation Risk for Internal Emitters, and U.K. Ministry of Defense
Oversight Committee on Depleted Uranium
christo@greenaudit.org

Leopoldo Caltagirone, Ph.D.
Chairman, Division of Biological Control, Berkeley, CA
lcbiocon@berkeley.edu

Liane Casten
Publisher, Chicago Media Watch, Chicago, IL
lcasten@sbcglobal.net

L. Terry Chappell, M.D.
President, The International College of Integrative Medicine, Bluffton, OH
terrychappell@blogspot.com

Richard Clapp, MPH, D.Sc.
Professor of Public Health, Boston University School of Public Health, Boston, MA
Member, Governing Board (Massachusetts) Alliance for a Healthy Tomorrow
richard.clapp@gmail.com

Gary Cohen
Executive Director, Environmental Health Fund, Jamaica Plain, MA
Director, Health Care Without Harm
gcohen@hcwh.org

Paul Connett, Ph.D.
Professor of Chemistry, St. Lawrence University, Canton, NY
President, Fluoride Action Network
paul@fluoridealert.org

Mary Cook
Managing Director, Occupational Health Clinics for Ontario Workers (OHCOW), Ontario, Canada
cook@*ohcow.on.ca*

Ronnie Cummins
National Director, Organic Consumers Association, Little Marais, MN
ronnie@organicconsumers.org

Alexandra Delinick, M.D.
Dean, School of Homeopathic Therapy, Vassil Levsky University, Sofia, Bulgaria
(Past, General Secretary, International Medical Homeopathic League)
homandgv@hol.gr

Lynn Ehrle, M.Ed.
Senior Research Fellow, CPC, Plymouth, MI
Vice President, Consumers Alliance of Michigan
ehrlebird@organicconsumers.org

Anwar Fazal
Chairperson, World Alliance for Breastfeeding Action
Senior Regional Advisor, the Urban Governance Initiative and United Nations Development Programme, Kuala Lumpur, Malaysia
Right Livelihood Award Laureate (The Alternative Nobel Prize)
(Former President, International Organization of Consumers Union)
anwarfazal2004@yahoo.com

Michael Green
Executive Director, Center for Environmental Health, Oakland, CA
ceh@cehca.org

Lennart Hardell, M.D., Ph.D.
Professor Epidemiology, University Hospital, Umea, Sweden
lennart.hardell@orebroll.se

James Huff, Ph.D.
National Institute of Environmental Health Sciences, Research Triangle Park, NC
huff1@niehs.nih.gov

Alison Linnecar
Coordinator, International Baby Food Action Network (IBFAN-GIFA)
Right Livelihood Award Laureate (The Alternative Nobel Prize)
alison.linnecar@gifa.org

Joseph Mangano, MPH, MBA
National Coordinator, Radiation and Public Health Project, Brooklyn, NY
odiejoe@aol.com

Elizabeth May
Director, Sierra Club of Canada, Ottawa, Canada
leader@greenparty.ca

Vicki Meyer, Ph.D.
Faculty, Women's Health, DePaul University, Chicago, IL
Founder, International Organization to Reclaim Menopause
vmeyer@depaul.edu

Raúl Montenegro, Ph.D.
Professor Evolutionary Biology, University Cordoba, Argentine
President, FUNAM (Foundation for Environmental Defense)
raulmontenegro@flash.com.ar

Vicente Navarro, M.D.
Professor of Health and Public Policy, The Johns Hopkins University, Baltimore, MD
Professor of Political and Social Sciences, Universitat Pompeu Fabra, Spain
Editor-in-Chief, International Journal of Health Services
vnavarro@jhsph.edu

Peter Orris, M.D., MPH
Professor, Occupational Medicine, University of Illinois Medical School, Chicago, IL
Professor, Internal and Preventive Medicine, Rush Medical College, Chicago, IL
Professor, Preventive Medicine, Northwestern University Feinberg School of Medicine, Chicago, IL
porris@uic.edu

Marjorie Roswell
Environmental activist, Baltimore, MD
mroswell@gmail.com

Janette Sherman, M.D.
Consultant Toxicologist, Alexandria, VA
Research Associate, Radiation and Public Health Project, NY
toxdoc.js@verizon.net

Ernest Sternglass, Ph.D.
Professor Emeritus, Department of Radiology, University of Pittsburgh, Pittsburgh, PA
erneststernglass@twcny.rr.com

Daniel Teitelbaum, M.D.
Professor, Preventive Medicine, University of Colorado, Denver, CO
toxdoc@ix.netcom.com

Stephen Tvedten, TIPM, CEI
Director, Institute of Pest Management, Inc., Marne, MI
stvedten@att.net

Jakob von Uexkull
President, Right Livelihood Award Foundation, Stockholm, Sweden
jakob@worldfuturecouncil.org

CARCINOGENIC INGREDIENTS IN COSMETICS AND TOILETRIES

FRANK CARCINOGENS

Benzyl Acetate*
Bisphenol A
Butyl Benzylphthalate
Butylated Hydroxyanisole (BHA)
Butylated Hydroxytoluene* (BHT)
"Coal Tar Dyes" (and Lakes)
    D & C
    Red 2, 3, 4, 8, 9, 10, 17, 19, & 33
    Green 5
    Orange 17
    FD & C
    Blue 1, 2 & 4
    Green 3
    Red 4 & 40
    Yellow 5 & 6
Diaminophenol
Diethanolamine (DEA)
DEA Oleamide Condensate
DEA Sodium Lauryl Sulfate
Diethylhexyl Phthalate

Dioctyl Adipate
Disperse Blue 1
Disperse Yellow 3
    Ethyl Alcohol
    Fluoride
Glutaral
Hydroquinone
Lead Acetate
Metheneamine
Methyl Methacrylate
Methylene Chloride
Mineral Spirits
Nitrofurazone
Nitrophenylenediamine
Phenyl-p-phenylenedediamine
Polyvinyl Pyrrolidone*
Pyrocatechol
Saccharin
Silica (crystalline)
Talc
Titanium Dioxide
Triethanolamine

---

*   Evidence is limited

GENTICALLY TOXIC (GENOTOXIC) CARCINOGENS

Aflatoxin
Arsenic
1,4-Dioxane
Ethylene Oxide
Formaldehyde
Lead
Nitrosodiethanolamine

HIDDEN CARCINOGENS

Contaminants

Acrylamide
Arsenic and lead, in coal tar dyes, polyvinyl acetate & PEG
Butadiene, in butane
Crystalline silica
DEA, in condensates & quaterniums
Ethylene oxide and dioxane
    Ceteareths
    Nonoxynol
    Octoxynol
    Oleths
    PEG
    Polysorbates
Ethylhexyl acrylate,
Formaldehyde
Organochlorine pesticides and PCBs, in lanolin
Polycyclic aromatic hydrocarbons, in petrolatum

Formaldehyde Precursors

Diazolidinyl Urea
DMDM-Hydantoin
Imidazolidinyl Urea
Metheneamine
Quaternium-15
Sodium/Hydroxymethylglycinate

Nitrosamine *Precursors*

    Bronopol
    Bromonidtrodioxane
    Diethanolamine (DEA)
    DEA-Cocmide, Lauramide & Oleamide condensates
    DEA-Sodium Lauryl Sulfate
    Metheneamine
    Morpholine
    Padimate-O
    Quaterniums
    Triethanolamine (TEA)